An Occupational Therapist's Guide to Sensory Integration and Adult Mental Health

of related interest

Nature-Based Allied Health Practice
Creative and Evidence-Based Strategies
Amy Wagenfeld and Shannon Marder
ISBN 978 1 80501 008 1
eISBN 978 1 80501 009 8

An Occupational Therapist's Guide to Sleep and Sleep Problems
Edited by Andrew Green and Cary Brown
Foreword by Michael Iwama
ISBN 978 1 84905 618 2
eISBN 978 1 78450 088 7

Occupational Therapy and Dementia
Promoting Inclusion, Rights and Opportunities for People Living With Dementia
Edited by Fiona Maclean, Alison Warren, Elaine Hunter and Lyn Westcott
Forewords by Scottish Dementia Working Group and Clare Hocking
ISBN 978 1 83997 062 7
eISBN 978 1 83997 061 0

An Occupational Therapist's Guide to
SENSORY INTEGRATION and ADULT MENTAL HEALTH

Rebecca Matson

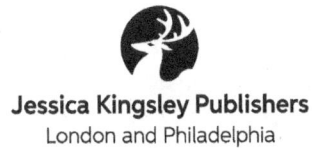

Jessica Kingsley Publishers
London and Philadelphia

First published in Great Britain in 2026 by Jessica Kingsley Publishers
An imprint of John Murray Press

Copyright © Rebecca Matson 2026

The right of Rebecca Matson to be identified as the Author of the Work has been asserted by her in accordance with the Copyright, Designs and Patents Act 1988.

Front cover image source: iStockphoto®/Shutterstock®. The cover image is for illustrative purposes only, and any person featuring is a model.

There are supplementary materials which can be downloaded from https://digitalhub.jkp.com/redeem using the code KWSHBDS for personal use with this programme but may not be reproduced for any other purposes without the permission of the publisher.

All rights reserved. No part of this publication may be reproduced, stored in a retrieval system, or transmitted, in any form or by any means without the prior written permission of the publisher, nor be otherwise circulated in any form of binding or cover other than that in which it is published and without a similar condition being imposed on the subsequent purchaser.

A CIP catalogue record for this title is available from the
British Library and the Library of Congress

ISBN 978 1 83997 914 9
eISBN 978 1 83997 915 6

Printed and bound in the United States by Integrated Books International

Jessica Kingsley Publishers' policy is to use papers that are natural, renewable and recyclable products and made from wood grown in sustainable forests. The logging and manufacturing processes are expected to conform to the environmental regulations of the country of origin.

Jessica Kingsley Publishers
Carmelite House
50 Victoria Embankment
London EC4Y 0DZ

www.jkp.com

John Murray Press
Part of Hodder & Stoughton Ltd
An Hachette Company

The authorised representative in the EEA is Hachette Ireland, 8 Castlecourt Centre, Dublin 15, D15 XTP3, Ireland (email: info@hbgi.ie)

Disclaimer

The information presented in this book is based on the authors' research, knowledge and clinical experience. It is intended for information purposes only and should not be considered a substitute for professional reasoning, clinical judgement or individualized risk assessment when implementing these ideas with your clients.

Readers are responsible for determining whether the strategies, techniques and resources discussed in this book are appropriate for specific client circumstances. The authors do not accept responsibility for any harm, loss or liability arising from the use or misuse of the material presented. While every effort has been made to ensure the accuracy of the information, healthcare practices are constantly evolving, and new knowledge may emerge that is not reflected in this publication. The authors disclaim any liability for errors, omissions or changes in the information presented.

Any references to external resources such as websites, textbooks or other materials are provided for information purposes only. The authors do not endorse or take responsibility for the content or accuracy of these external sources.

Contents

1. Introduction.................................... 9
   Rebecca Matson

2. Psychotic Disorders 15
   Leanne Duggan and Rebecca Matson

3. Borderline Personality Disorder 31
   Rebecca Matson

4. Eating Disorders 45
   Rebecca Matson

5. PTSD/Trauma.................................. 59
   Rebecca Matson

6. Affective and Anxiety Disorders 72
   Leanne Duggan and Rebecca Matson

7. Dementia...................................... 91
   Leanne Duggan and Rebecca Matson

8. Assessment and Goal Setting................... 113
   Leanne Duggan and Rebecca Matson

9. Levels of Intervention 138
   Rebecca Matson

10. Sensory Strategies 147
    Rebecca Matson

11. Sensory-Informed Approaches................. 160
    Rebecca Matson

12. Ayres Sensory Integration®. 168
    Rebecca Matson

13. Outcome Measurement 184
    Rebecca Matson

    APPENDIX 1: SENSORY ASSESSMENT REPORT TEMPLATE 196

    APPENDIX 2: SENSORY SUPPORT PLAN TEMPLATE. 199

    APPENDIX 3: SENSORY GROUP PROGRAMME 201

    APPENDIX 4: TRAINING SESSION POWERPOINT 218

    REFERENCES 232

    SUBJECT INDEX. 248

    AUTHOR INDEX 254

CHAPTER 1

Introduction

REBECCA MATSON

When I started my journey into using sensory approaches in mental health there were very few resources available, as well as very little published research focused on this specific field of practice. I was fortunate to be able to form links with others working in similar fields while completing my sensory integration training, and also to have guidance from an experienced mentor during the end stages, but found myself searching for resources to support my practice and help me to consider how best to approach working with my clients. The idea for this book came from a desire to create a resource I wish I'd had to guide me when starting out, and I hope this book will meet at least part of this need for you. The use of sensory approaches of varying levels is rapidly increasing within mental health settings, along with a steady increase in the evidence base. As occupational therapists a central part of our practice is ensuring we integrate evidence-based practice in all that we do, so it is essential we remain aware of these developments.

Aim of the book

The aim of this book is to meet a dual need: to bring together current evidence and thinking on using sensory approaches with different client groups; and to provide you with practical ideas and resources to support your day-to-day practice. For this reason the book is separated first into chapters according to diagnostic groups to enable you to reflect on the needs of your client group and navigate to the sections that may be most useful to you. While as occupational therapists we often try to move away from diagnostic frameworks, much of the evidence is focused in this way, and also there will be some commonality in approaches that can be considered. The second half of the book is structured according to stages of the process you are likely to follow in working with individuals considering assessment approaches and priorities which then inform goal setting; intervention and, more specifically, the different levels of intervention used within sensory integration according to need and clinician training, including sensory strategies, sensory-based interventions and Ayres Sensory Integration® (ASI®); and lastly a chapter considering outcome measurement.

Why consider sensory in mental health?

A number of you are likely to be reading this book as you are already convinced of the need to 'think sensory' when working in mental health, whereas others may be less convinced, and some may think there is a need but not understand exactly why. The first and primary rationale for thinking this way is that we are all sensory beings with our own particular sensory needs and preferences that make us who we are, and shape our lives, potentially impacting on areas such as our choice of friends, our career, where we live and the hobbies we choose. Think about what you do to unwind after a long day, whether that is to spend time in the gym, go for a walk, or have a bath. Most likely you do this for the sensory benefits it gives you. Much of what we do is influenced by our sensory preferences but without us being consciously aware of how much of a factor this is. As Dunn (2001, p. 608) advocates, 'Sensory processing patterns are reflections of who we are: these patterns are not a pathology that needs fixing.'

Always keep that in mind, and view sensory patterns as an area that enables us to better understand and work with our clients, rather than another symptom or problem to add to the list.

The second reason to consider sensory approaches in mental health is that sensory processing is foundational to everything we do, and to higher-level skills such as emotional regulation, communication and reasoning (Ayres, 1979; Bundy & Lane, 2020), all of which are important in supporting our wellbeing and mental health. If we are not able to effectively process sensory input at a foundational level this will impact on various areas of our occupational performance and occupational identity. When working with any client group to enable them to maximize their occupational performance, consideration needs to be given to sensory processing and how this may be part of the picture both in the barriers they face, but also in the factors that could be used to enable participation and wellbeing. Whatever our clients' goals and aspirations there are likely to be areas of sensory processing we can either nurture or support them with to enable their success.

The third and final reason I want to highlight here is the collaborative and empowering nature of sensory approaches that tends to be so different to other approaches commonly used within mental health, which are much more therapist-led, placing the therapist as the expert and the one in control (Dempsey, 2016; Williamson & Ennals, 2020). Sensory approaches within mental health are by nature more levelling as the client is the expert of their own sensory needs, with you, as the therapist, acting as a guide supporting them in their journey to increase their understanding and ability to regulate their responses. This is not to say that using sensory approaches does not require expertise from you as a therapist, but even when working at what would be considered the highest level of sensory intervention, Ayres Sensory Integration, where fidelity is a primary consideration, intervention remains client-led with fidelity principles focused on elements such as collaborating in activity choice and supporting their intrinsic motivation (Schaaf & Mailloux, 2015). Being able to help someone to have a greater understanding of their own sensory processing patterns is something I have found to be such an empowering experience for those I worked with, as well as one that has often given them answers to experiences they have had for years but without knowing why. It has helped to normalize and explain difficulties someone may have been having or their reactions to different situations. One client who will always stick with me shared how others often thought she was drunk or careless due to the frequency with which she would stumble, trip or bump into things. Completing a sensory assessment revealed sensory integration and praxis challenges that explained these difficulties. Giving her the words to be able to explain why this was happening and relating it to the differences in her sensory processing patterns led to an immediate shift in her perception of herself and her confidence in responding to others. This is just one such experience that has fostered my passion for sensory integration in mental health over the years and a big part of why I hope this book inspires others to do the same.

The relevance of sensory approaches in mental health

While above I have asserted the importance of seeing sensory processing patterns as part of who someone is, rather than an issue or an area to be remedied, a significant reason to advocate for sensory approaches is the evidence for altered sensory processing patterns that have been identified as happening in the context of different mental health conditions. This is the reason why within each of the condition-specific chapters there is a discussion of commonly noted sensory processing patterns or needs. While as occupational therapists we often pride ourselves in working outside of a medical model there is merit in being able to engage with this dialogue both in advocating for resources and in reframing the responses and interactions of our clients to other professionals who might also be working with them. Providing an understanding of someone's sensory responses can help to provide a new lens for what may to others appear to be unreasonable or behavioural responses.

Consider that person who may seem to suddenly become agitated out of nowhere and perhaps begins shouting at someone to move away. The reaction may appear incongruous to those around them, but could actually be a response to something others barely notice, like a slight brush as someone walks past them. For an individual with a heightened sensitivity to touch, an apparently small trigger like this could cause them to go into a hyper-alert state. Or consider that individual who is seen as being lazy or not motivated for change due to declining opportunities to go different places, but when they do go out become quickly overwhelmed by the noises, lights and bustle of people and so has learnt it is safer to avoid such situations.

The evidence base for the prevalence of sensory processing needs within mental health is steadily increasing, much of which is summarized in the proceeding chapters of this book. Sensory processing patterns and mental health needs can be seen as a 'chicken and egg' situation, as I often think it is difficult to see which preceded the other. There is a bidirectional relationship between our arousal levels and sensory response, with those who experience increased sensory responsivity being more prone to fluctuations in mood and regulation, and those with difficulties regulating their mood being more prone to experience increased sensory responsivity. Think of how many people, when anxious, become more easily agitated by sensory inputs such as background noise or bright lighting which they may usually tolerate, but how if you have an increased sensitivity to a certain sensory input such as touch or sound then encountering higher levels or unexpected input may cause you to become anxious or agitated in response. Or consider someone who has experienced difficulties with their motor coordination or planning since childhood and the frustration they may have experienced in everyday tasks, or the negative responses they may have received from others, and the impact this is likely to have had on their wellbeing. There are a number of other factors involved in whether experiencing such challenges is likely to lead to mental health difficulties, but hopefully you can see how they could become a part of the process. I worked with several people over the years where I wondered if their life may have been very different if they had been able to access the support they needed in these areas when a child.

Implications of sensory processing needs

As occupational therapists our primary concern when working with people is enabling occupational participation and engagement; even when working from what is often known as more of a 'bottom up' approach in relation to underlying sensory processing, we should always be doing so with a view of the overarching occupational needs of that individual. Sensory processing challenges will impact on different areas of an individual's functioning, and understanding this central component is integral to effectively working with someone. However, we need to keep in view that sensory processing would fit within the area of underlying performance components in Hocking's (2001) widely accepted conceptual framework for occupation-based assessment, and see these areas as components of an individual's occupational performance. In this framework the meaning an occupation holds for an individual and how it shapes their occupational identity is at the top; followed by the purpose of that occupation in their life; the form or the way in which that occupation is carried out; and lastly the performance components that are relevant to understand the barriers to occupational performance that person is experiencing. When identifying occupational challenges and strengths we need to not only understand how someone's sensory processing may have altered, but also how this connects to their occupational life and being able to do what they need to or want to do.

Ensuring that we work in this way is an important part of protecting the philosophy of our profession as well as retaining a meaningful person-centred focus within the process of working with each individual. The extent to which an individual's sensory processing challenges will have impacted on their occupations and their wellbeing will vary from person to person, even if they experience the same underlying difficulties, and it is this that will inform priorities for intervention and even whether intervention is considered of importance. Adults in particular tend to have experienced these difficulties for a number of years and have learnt alternative ways to complete activities, or adapted to the difficulties they cause, and may not want to or see a need to change this. If we solely see the sensory processing challenges without putting them in the context of someone's life we run the risk of adding additional demands or priorities onto our clients that they do not want.

Sensory cues from within the environment are also a highly important part of successful engagement in occupations and hold particular relevance for mental health. Bailliard (2015) discusses the impact of what he terms sensory dissonance on mental health, where the sensory cues from our environment do not fit with those expected or needed. A number of the individuals we work with in mental health spend periods within inpatient services where they have little control over the sensory cues related to their day-to-day occupations, and we need to consider the impact of that on their performance when working with them. Another way in which this is of relevance is when an individual changes their living environment or work role and is required to adjust to a new environment which may have very different sensory elements. For those we work with who experience challenges in sensory processing this is likely to hold particular relevance.

How to approach this book

This book is structured so you can move between different sections of relevance to you or relating to the queries you may have. Chapters 2–7 relate to different conditions and provide you with an overview of the literature, sensory processing patterns that might be seen, the functional impacts of these patterns, and approaches to assessment and intervention when working with that client group. While elements of sensory strategies are included within these chapters the focus is on considerations and variations specific to each client group. Broader guidance relating to the development of sensory plans and kits is included within Chapter 10, Sensory Strategies, as the information within this chapter is likely to be of use for any client in supporting overall improved self-regulation. Chapters 8–13 focus on different stages of the occupational therapy process, including the different levels of intervention, and provide you with ideas of how to approach these different stages and what you might need to know when deciding on your intervention approach, for example when different approaches may be relevant and what level of training is required in order to use them. The final section contains appendices of practical resources for practice including a sensory assessment report template, a sensory support plan template, a sensory group programme and a training session template. All pages marked with ✶ can be downloaded from https://digitalhub.jkp.com/ redeem using the code: KWSHBDS

I hope this book will become a resource that supports you in your ongoing journey and development that you are able to come back to again and again.

CHAPTER 2

Psychotic Disorders

LEANNE DUGGAN AND REBECCA MATSON

Psychosis can be a feature of a number of mental health conditions, but the most frequently connected conditions include:

- first episode psychosis
- schizophrenia
- schizoaffective disorder.

Therefore, much of the discussion in this chapter will relate to these disorders. Experience of psychosis may include hallucinations, delusions and thought disturbances and tends to have a significant impact on an individual's ability to engage in valued occupations and their overall wellbeing. While psychosis can also be a feature in other conditions such as bipolar disorder, these conditions are considered elsewhere in this book.

Psychotic disorders are generally diagnosed if a client presents with a combination of positive and negative symptoms shown in Table 2.1.

Table 2.1 Positive and negative symptoms of psychosis (American Psychiatric Association (APA), 2013; Health and Safety Executive (HSE), 2019; NHS, 2023)

Positive symptoms	Negative symptoms
Hallucinations	Low mood
Delusions	Avolition
Paranoia	Social withdrawal
Thought disorder	Cognitive changes (e.g. decreased concentration)

Psychotic disorders can be described as having three distinct phases:

- **Prodromal phase:** This encompasses the development of a number of non-specific behavioural, mental and emotional changes including decreased motivation, increased social isolation and feelings of anxiety or worry (French et al., 2010). This phase only occurs before the first episode of psychosis.
- **Acute phase:** Active symptoms such as alterations in sensory perception (hallucinations), altered beliefs (delusions), feelings of paranoia, and suspiciousness (Hughes, 2010).
- **Recovery phase:** Symptoms abate and the person experiences a gradual return to function (Brown, 2011; French et al., 2010).

Where more than one episode of psychosis occurs, the individual experiences a relapse of symptoms, returning to the acute phase of illness (French et al., 2010). Further episodes result in a cycle between the acute and recovery phases of psychosis, which is characteristic of clients with a diagnosis of schizoaffective disorder and schizophrenia. Consideration of how a client's ability to process sensation may alter in connection with the phase of illness will help inform an approach to intervention best suited to their presenting needs.

Categories of psychotic disorders

As 'psychosis' is a broad term, encompassing a range of disorders, it is useful to identify how the most common forms of the disorder are identified:

- **First episode psychosis** is typically described as the emergence of moderately severe psychotic symptoms for a minimum period of seven consecutive days (HSE, 2019).
- **Schizophrenia** is characterized by recurrent episodes of illness, whereby the client experiences a number of acute episodes, resulting in a significant impact on their cognition and functioning (HSE, 2019; NHS, 2023).
- **Schizoaffective disorder** features additional considerations which encompass an affective element, resulting in substantial fluctuations in mood (APA, 2013).

Each of these conditions tend to have a significant impact on daily functioning and quality of life, highlighting an important role for occupational therapists. Psychotic symptoms experienced as part of these conditions influence the perception and regulation of sensory input, presenting challenges to both function and participation in occupation (Halperin & Falk-Kessler, 2020; Lipskaya-Velikovsky et al., 2015). A number of the particular areas in which this is evident will be reviewed within this chapter.

Alterations in sensory processing
Neurological threshold

Individuals experiencing psychosis have been found to demonstrate a pattern of sensory responsivity that is similar to other mental health conditions, but distinct from the general population. An early study by Brown et al. (2002) using the Adolescent/Adult Sensory Profile (Brown & Dunn, 2002) suggested individuals with schizophrenia showed a pattern of higher levels of sensation avoiding (i.e. a low threshold for sensory input and an active response to manage this) and low registration (i.e. high threshold for sensory input and passive response), alongside reduced levels of sensation seeking, a pattern that has been further confirmed by more recent studies but with evidence of the sensory sensitivity pattern also being apparent (Halperin & Falk-Kessler, 2020; Parham et al., 2019; Pfeiffer et al., 2014). This pattern appears to be consistent amongst both those diagnosed with a psychotic disorder and those considered at high risk of developing psychosis, suggesting the prevalence of ongoing sensory modulation challenges within this population. Lipskaya-Velikovsky et al. (2015), however, identified low registration to be the only pattern that was significantly higher in an inpatient population with schizophrenia than the general population, but with no correlation between this pattern and symptoms of illness or participation challenges experienced. They suggest that this may be due to the under-responsivity having predated the onset of schizophrenia, potentially impacting on progression of the cognitive and emotional aspects of the condition.

Parham et al. (2019) also propose that differences in sensory modulation could be a potential early indicator or factor in the development of psychosis. Their study used the Adolescent/Adult Sensory Profile (Brown & Dunn, 2002) to identify the presence of sensory modulation challenges across two groups in comparison to normative data: those at clinical high risk of psychosis and those at low risk of psychosis. The clinical high-risk group echoed the pattern of modulation difficulties seen in previous studies of those with psychosis, showing heightened levels of sensory avoidance, sensory sensitivity and low registration with decreased levels of sensation seeking. This was a significant difference to the low-risk group, who only showed reduced levels of sensation seeking in comparison to norms. Parham et al. (2019) suggest these sensory differences may act as a marker for transition to the acute stage of psychosis and could inform intervention to remediate the impact of these difficulties.

Developing an increased understanding of how sensory processing is altered in both those at risk of developing psychosis and those with long-term psychotic disorders has potential clinical significance in informing improved ways of working in view of both environmental supports and therapeutic engagement (Halperin & Falk-Kessler, 2020; Parham et al., 2019).

Underlying neuroscience considerations

Similar to other psychiatric conditions, dysregulation of the hypothalamic–pituitary–adrenal (HPA) axis and resultant increased cortisol levels has been suggested to be a significant factor in stress responses within schizophrenia as well as in the cognitive decline that is often experienced (Cherian et al., 2019). The HPA axis involves the release of a chain of activating hormones from the hypothalamus, pituitary gland and adrenal gland, which ultimately results in the release of cortisol (Bear et al., 2020). Further discussion of the role of the HPA axis and its relationship to modulation of arousal is included in Chapter 6, Affective and Anxiety Disorders.

A potential contributor to this HPA axis dysregulation is the experience of childhood trauma, which has been identified as a risk factor for the development of psychosis and suggested to increase the severity of perceptual disturbances, affective symptoms and functional impairments (Giannopoulou et al., 2023; Lowey et al., 2019). Clients with a diagnosis of schizophrenia are 2.72 times more likely to have had adverse experiences in childhood than the general population (Varese et al., 2012). These traumatic experiences lead to increased levels of sensitization and activation of the HPA axis, with subsequent activation of the sympathetic nervous system and increased safety-seeking responses (Murphy et al., 2022). Multiple traumatic occurrences increase the likelihood of someone considered at clinical high risk of developing psychosis, transitioning to acute psychosis (Giannopoulou et al., 2023).

Another potential factor is dysconnectivity of the thalamus, which has been suggested to precede the onset of psychosis, impacting on regulation of the HPA axis (Cherian et al., 2019; Parham et al., 2019). This dysfunction of the thalamus has been connected to both sensory motor impacts and the development of delusions (Crail-Melendez et al., 2013; Parham et al., 2019). The avoidant response often seen in someone experiencing psychosis in relation to sensory input is likely to be connected to this HPA axis dysregulation and an attempt to reduce the level of perceived threat experienced due to being in a state of hyper-arousal. However, the connection between the apparently contrasting responses to sensory input of hyper- and hypo-responsivity in those with psychotic disorders may have quite a different aetiology to that seen in other psychiatric conditions such as borderline personality disorder where the experience of low registration has been suggested to be a result of overwhelm followed by shutdown to manage hyper-reactivity. Brown et al. (2002) suggest instead that this apparently contradictory pattern of mixed responsivity corresponds with suggestions by Cromwell (1993) that individuals with schizophrenia simultaneously experience what he termed 'super sensitivity' and 'over-inhibition' of sensory input. This is thought to result in limited initial registration of sensory input leading to missing information to inform responses, but then once sensory input is registered it is rapidly perceived as a threat, resulting in an avoidant safety response. This dysregulation has also been suggested to lead to high levels of cognitive impairment due to reductions in the volume of the prefrontal cortex and decreased dopamine activity (Mikulska et al., 2021).

Broader differences in sensory processing in schizophrenia have also been connected specifically with the thalamus due to its central role in the process of sensory gating, and therefore filtering of information, to ensure that only necessary information proceeds to higher processing areas within the brain (Anticevic et al., 2015; Crail-Melendez et al., 2013). In addition to the variable responsivity to sensory input discussed above, alterations in the thalamus also impact on the process of sensory discrimination, with ineffective filtering impacting on the ability to identify the qualities of sensory input needed to inform this process. In contrast with this reduced activity, a hyper-connectivity between the thalamus and sensory motor areas within the cortex has been suggested, creating the potential for excessive motor responses to sensory input, which may be evident in the presentation of sensory avoidance suggested to be a feature of psychosis (Anticevic et al., 2015; Parham et al., 2019). These changes are outlined in Figure 2.1.

Other specific areas in the brain connected with altered sensory processing include the prefrontal cortex, amygdala and the hippocampus. The prefrontal cortex is thought to be impaired in its role of top-down inhibition of response to sensory input and therefore responsivity is more easily triggered (Bear et al., 2020). Alongside this an individual is thought to experience heightened reactivity of the amygdala due to a reduction in hippocampal volume, resulting in an inability to regulate their reactivity and a more extreme response to sensory input once fully registered (Mikulska et al., 2021).

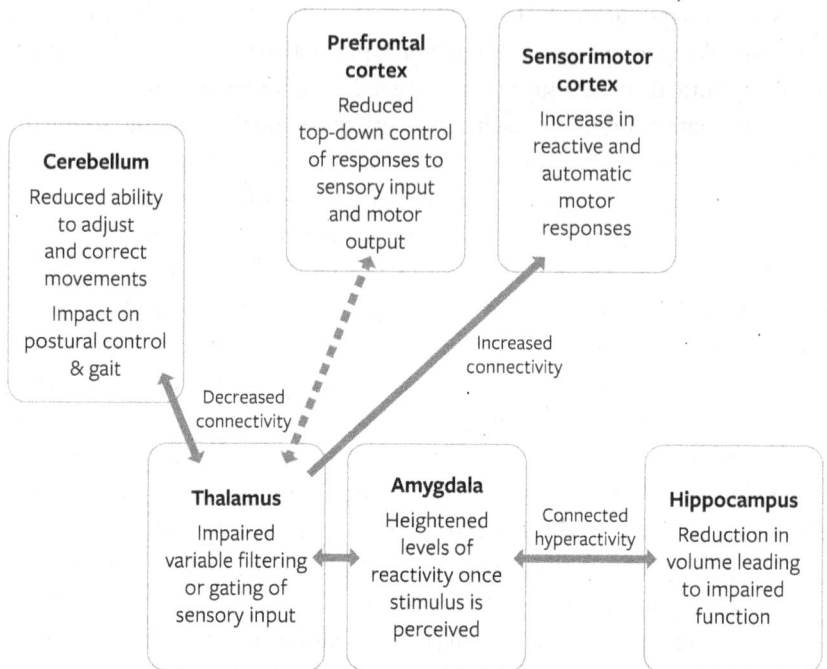

Figure 2.1 Areas of the brain impacted in schizophrenia that are connected with sensory processing and motor control (Anticevic et al., 2015; Crail-Melendez et al., 2013; Mikulska et al., 2021)

Differences in specific sensory systems

The sensory systems that have received the most attention within the literature relating to psychosis are the auditory and visual systems. Difficulties within these systems are thought to relate both to regulation of these inputs and discriminative ability (Ramsay et al., 2020; Sanchis-Asensi et al., 2022). Alterations within these senses have been suggested to occur in relation to the experience of psychosis rather than specific diagnoses such as schizophrenia or bipolar, but with the greatest level of impairment evident in schizophrenia (Ramsay et al., 2020). There has also been some suggestion of impairments within the tactile system that have been found to impact on a sense of connection to the body as well as lead to reduced pain perception (Costantini et al., 2020; Vaughan et al., 2019). This suggests that alterations within the tactile system relate primarily to its discriminative ability rather than modulation of the input.

While hallucinatory experiences can relate to auditory, visual, somatosensory, olfactory and gustatory input the most frequently experienced is auditory hallucinations, and therefore it is perhaps to be expected that individuals experiencing psychosis will show altered responsivity within this system (Horga &

Abi-Dargham, 2019). Low registration or under-responsivity in auditory processing has been found to be the greatest area of difference between individuals with schizophrenia and both those with other psychiatric diagnoses and the general population (Harrison et al., 2019; Sanchis-Asensi et al., 2022). This area of difficulty was also found to have the highest correlation with lower quality of life in a study by Sanchis-Asensi et al. (2022), making it an important area for consideration and intervention.

A study by Carter et al. (2017) found evidence that the difficulties with processing within the visual and auditory systems related to higher-level cortical processing and integration rather than the initial perception of the sensory information through the receptors. The results of their study suggested that the level of difficulty experienced correlates with the severity of positive symptoms (Carter et al., 2017). A possible rationale for this is impairments in the process of cortical inhibition resulting from a trauma response to the sensory input, which is too readily perceived as a potential threat.

Motor planning

King (1974) first suggested the sensory integrative basis to the motor planning and postural deficits often seen in psychotic disorders. She suggests that deficits in proprioceptive processing result in impairment in the integration of the senses that is required to inform praxis. However, since this study much of the published literature in relation to psychotic disorders has focused on sensory modulation, with only a small number considering the motor planning difficulties suggested by King. The results of these studies are considered below.

Halperin and Falk-Kessler (2020) used the Assessment of Motor and Process Skills (AMPS) (Fisher, 2010) to evaluate the correlation between sensory processing patterns and altered motor and processing skills in individuals with schizophrenia spectrum disorders (SSD). They found a potential correlation between sensation avoiding and motor deficits and a correlation between sensory avoiding and process skills. This suggests that individuals with schizophrenia may experience impairments within multiple aspects of praxis, including not only the ability to execute a movement but also earlier stages, including developing the initial idea and identifying a plan to execute the motor pattern. They suggest that impairments in motor planning are more prevalent amongst individuals with schizophrenia than those with other mental health conditions.

How much of these impairments are connected to alterations in sensory processing is unclear; however, there has been some suggestion that heightened difficulties with visual motor integration correlate with increased levels of positive symptoms in those with schizophrenia (Carter et al., 2017). This is inclusive of difficulties with visual tracking and visual discrimination, both of which hold importance in providing the necessary information to inform motor skills and balance control. Corresponding difficulties have also been identified in clients with other psychotic disorders (Bailliard & Whigham, 2017; Feldman et al., 2020; Ramsey et al., 2020). Similar to the earlier study by King (1974), Harrison et al. (2019) found individuals with schizophrenia have reduced proprioception, impacting negatively on body awareness, motor planning and gait.

Postural differences, specifically hyperlordosis, have also been identified as a common occurrence in schizophrenia as well as impaired balance and ataxic gait (Feldman et al., 2020). These differences are thought to relate primarily to alterations in executive function and the changes in the basal ganglia, thalamus and cerebellum that are associated with schizophrenia. However, the impact of reduced visual discrimination has also been suggested as a potential causal factor, leading to increased reliance on the other senses that inform postural control (Ramsay et al., 2020). Overall this is an area that requires further investigation to gain a more complete picture of how praxis skills may be altered in psychotic disorders and impact on occupational performance as a result.

Impact of sensory processing on functioning

Evidence in relation to the impact of sensory processing differences on functioning for this client group is limited overall, but there has been some suggestion of specific areas of impact, including social and cognitive functioning. A significant barrier in relation to social functioning and development of relationships is the difficulty commonly experienced with visual discrimination, which has been suggested to relate most strongly to facial recognition and interpretation of expressions (Osborne et al., 2022). This is likely to lead to difficulties forming positive relationships due to impaired reading of social cues and difficulties with resultant reciprocal interactions. Alongside this, altered perception of verbal tone has also been suggested to impact on levels of social participation (Bailliard & Whigham, 2017; Sanchis-Asensi et al., 2022).

Difficulties with auditory and visual processing have been connected with both work performance and community integration (Sanchis-Asensi et al., 2022). Correlations have also been suggested between sensory processing patterns and quality of life, with lower scores on sensation seeking being connected with a greater pattern of withdrawal and higher levels of avoidance, resulting in a more sedentary lifestyle (Good et al., 2010). Greater levels of both low registration and sensory sensitivity have also shown a moderate level of correlation with decreased psychological health (Sanchis-Asensi et al., 2022).

Difficulties with sensory gating, that is, the filtering of sensory input to ensure only relevant or necessary sensory input is attended to, have been linked to both cognitive difficulties and increased distraction when completing daily tasks (Champagne & Pfeiffer, 2020; Javitt & Freedman, 2015). These cognitive impairments alongside sensory processing difficulties have been found to significantly alter levels of independent functioning for those experiencing psychosis, including activities important to sustain independent living such as cooking as well as participation in wider activities in their local community. Therefore, occupational therapy intervention has a central role in early intervention services in particular to assess the extent of the barriers, and mitigate this impact in order to facilitate meaningful engagement (Thomas et al., 2022).

A sensory lens on hallucinations

Hallucinations can be described as sensory experiences outside of an individual's control that are experienced as real by them but lack support from external sensory inputs (Pezzoli & Venneri, 2021). The experience of hallucinations is one of the primary distinguishing features of psychosis and can also cause high levels of distress and mistrust in both those around the person and their physical environment. Hallucinations can take many different sensory forms, and while the most commonly experienced and acknowledged are auditory hallucinations, they are also known to occur within the visual, somatosensory, olfactory and gustatory systems, as is noted above (Horga & Abi-Dargham, 2019). During the experience of auditory hallucinations increased levels of activation of areas of the brain connected with speech rather than auditory processing have been noted, including the anterior cingulate cortex, cerebellum and right superior temporal pole (Pezzoli & Venneri, 2021).

These differences, alongside reduced connectivity between the cerebellum and the prefrontal cortex, have been connected to the experience of delusions due to the impact they have on the evaluation of sensory input against prior experiences (Anticevic et al., 2015; Crail-Melendez et al., 2013). Comparison of sensory input against prior experiences is vital in prioritizing how we should respond and evaluating factors such as our safety in this context. Difficulty in doing this is therefore likely to result in an unnecessary heightened threat response to innocuous sensory inputs.

The intensity of experience of auditory hallucinations has been connected with the impairments in P50 gating that are evident in schizophrenia (Javitt & Freedman, 2015). Javitt and Freedman (2015) suggest two main reasons for this: if an individual is unable to fully register simple sensory information this will have an impact on their ability to ascertain its significance, and neuronal impairments in sensory regions are also likely to be present in connected areas for executive functioning. This leads to heightened difficulties in comparing sensory input to prior experiences, or other sensory references that may support ability to challenge hallucinatory experiences through assessing their origin and qualities.

Considerations for assessment and intervention
Approaches to assessment

Individuals experiencing psychosis are likely to experience high levels of confusion and potential mistrust of the sensory information they are receiving due to factors such as hallucinatory sensory experiences, which they are constantly having to challenge. This will need to be kept in consideration during both the assessment and intervention process. There is also the potential for red herrings to have a particular impact when completing self-report assessments due to unusual sensory experiences, and this may need to be accounted for when choosing which sensory assessments to use. For example, an individual may report becoming dizzy easily but this could be the result of medication side effects rather than altered vestibular processing. Or they may need to ask others to repeat what they say because of the distraction of auditory hallucinations, rather than an under-responsivity to auditory input.

The Adolescent/Adult Sensory Profile (Brown & Dunn, 2002) has been used in studies with individuals experiencing psychosis, suggesting it has a reasonable level of reliability with this client group. In the studies both by Brown et al. (2002) and Sanchis-Asensi et al. (2022) participants were described as relatively clinically stable, therefore the same level of reliability in self-report could not necessarily be assumed when using with those in a more acute phase of illness. There may also need to be consideration of the fact that sensory reactivity may alter as symptoms of psychosis decrease and therefore reassessment may be needed and review of any sensory strategies put in place.

Sensory processing alterations have been suggested to extend beyond solely modulation difficulties, therefore it may be best to complete an assessment that also considers additional areas such as discrimination and praxis. The Adult/Adolescent Sensory History (May-Benson, 2015) or the Sensory Processing Measure, Second Edition (SPM-2) (Parham et al., 2021) may be appropriate choices for this to gain insight into sensory processing challenges. Each of these assessments also have carer/observer versions which allow for adjustment in approach for those in more acute phases of illness who may struggle to reliably self-report. Further potential assessment choices are discussed within Chapter 8, Assessment and Goal Setting.

Approaches to intervention

Sensory intervention that is reflective of the client's stage of illness may be focused on areas such as grounding strategies to support improved concentration and regulation, strategies to help counter or provide distraction during hallucinatory experiences, or to increase arousal levels when experiencing negative symptoms of schizophrenia. The overarching aim of intervention may be directly influenced by their stage of illness. For example, in the acute phase the therapeutic focus may be on reduction of distress, while the recovery phase may require an approach that is more tailored to meet the client's specific sensory needs in order to promote function and engagement in meaningful occupations.

Development of a sensory plan can be helpful to provide strategies that can be used at different times to support maintenance of arousal levels and engagement in valued activities. Chapter 10, Sensory Strategies, provides guidance on the broader use of sensory plans and kits that may be beneficial alongside the information within this chapter. Depending on the difficulties identified, it may be appropriate to consider more focused Ayres Sensory Integration (ASI) intervention, which is discussed in Chapter 12, Ayres Sensory Integration®, as many of the considerations into how this might be carried out would carry across the different diagnoses discussed. Therefore, the focus below is on approaches or strategies that may be of benefit to all. Where an individual has experienced trauma and shows safety-seeking behaviours, intervention priorities should consider the following areas:

- reducing their level of arousal using strategies that are down-regulating
- promotion of feelings of safety through interventions and strategies that provide a grounding sensation
- altering physical environments to promote feelings of safety and to increase functional capacity
- providing education on how their sensory processing is influencing behaviour to the client and their families, where appropriate.

Using a sensory-informed approach with clients with a diagnosis of psychosis who have experienced trauma allows for the provision of a non-pharmacological method of reducing distress and empowering them to actively engage in their own recovery.

Note: It is important to ascertain if the client has an experience of trauma when considering ideas for intervention. This is an important component to add into your clinical reasoning, to ensure therapeutic safety throughout your assessment and intervention process. If the client demonstrates or subjectively reports discomfort or features of distress when trialling any of the strategies, their use is to be discontinued.

You should also check for the presence of allergies, asthma or hay fever that could be exacerbated by different scents, for example, or sensitivity to products such as talcum powder that can be present on items such as Theraband. Retaining the manufacturer instructions provided with any equipment is important to support this.

Strategies and approaches

Sensory strategies can be used to help an individual feel more grounded and present but also to divert attention away from problematic stimuli or distressing experiences such as hallucinations. This can be achieved in a number of ways, and it is likely to take trial and error to identify those that are most effective for each individual. Each section below contains a list of ideas.

Strategies to support grounding

- Scented oils or products can be highly grounding and help to divert attention away from distressing or distracting experiences.
    - Be aware of the strong emotional connection smells can have; caution is needed when initially trialling these. Use of a new scent should not be first trialled with an individual in a distress state.
    - Use of scents often serves as a temporary measure of distraction, which will create an opportunity to follow up with more targeted strategy use.
- Biting into a lemon or sucking on a sour sweet or strong mint.
- Using a spiky massage ball. Experiment with rolling it over different body parts to alter the intensity of input.
- Holding an ice cube or ice pack.
- Using weighted items such as a weighted shawl.
- Using a night light/projector can be helpful to provide diverting visual stimuli.

- Doing wall or chair push-ups provides strong proprioceptive input that helps the person feel present in their body.
- Yoga poses with a high level of muscle stretch. This can be increased further through the use of yoga blocks.
- Holding a textured pebble or shell can provide grounding tactile input.

Strategies to increase arousal and support concentration

- White noise can help divert attention from other distracting background noises.
- Alerting smells such as citrus, mint or eucalyptus.
- Chewing gum or chewy sweets.
- Sitting on a gym ball or wobble cushion can provide regulating inputs.
- Using fidget tools such as tangle fidgets or stress balls.
- Taking a cold shower.
- Creating movement breaks in activities requiring longer periods of concentration.
- Drinking through a straw.
- Sucking on sour sweets or strong mints.

Strategies to support body awareness

Improving body awareness can both facilitate a grounded state and support development of improved motor planning. The strategies below focus primarily on provision of proprioceptive, vestibular and tactile feedback. Using your skills of activity analysis, you can adjust these to match with individual interests and activities for each individual.

- Gardening activities that involve heavy muscle work such as digging.
- Holding a plank or doing wall or chair press-ups.
- Wearing compression or Lycra garments.
- Using wrist or ankle weights to increase proprioceptive feedback during activities such as walking.
- Resistance band exercises.
- Yoga exercises and poses.
- Weight training.
- Swimming.

Strategies for distraction

While not a longer-term solution, it may be that diversional strategies are needed in the moment to help reduce levels of immediate distress. This could be as a distraction or a way to support the challenging of hallucinatory experiences. Below are some ideas for doing this:

- Using a fibre optic lamp, night light or projector.
- Aromatherapy oils or scented products can provide a diversion from olfactory hallucinations.
  - Alerting scents, such as citrus or mint, are likely to be most effective.
  - It is worthwhile exploring both pleasant and noxious sources of olfactory stimulation to identify which provides an adequate level of distraction.
- Listening to a white noise app or preferred music.
- Biting into a lemon or sucking on a sour sweet can support grounding and diversion.
- Holding onto an ice cube or ice pack.
- Using fidget tools can help someone feel present and divert attention from hallucinatory experiences.
- Using colouring books or puzzles can help to engage attention.
- Opportunities for movement to enhance vestibular and proprioceptive input (e.g. dancing, home exercise programme).

CASE STUDY – Jaxon
Background

Jaxon, aged 20, was referred to occupational therapy services as part of his treatment with the first episode psychosis (FEP) team. The referral identified that his psychotic symptoms had mostly resolved, but that he was having extreme difficulty completing his college assignments and was about to lose his place on his course. During the initial interview Jaxon reported working for hours each day, but finding he could not remember any of the content, so he would repeat the same content the following day – which negatively impacted on his progression. He reported feeling well from a mental-state perspective, but at times he would become highly distressed as he felt something was crawling over his skin when on public transport. Further exploration of this revealed that this occurred when the train moved at speed, and this had led to him avoiding public transport apart from attending his appointments with the FEP team.

Assessment and formulation of difficulties

Completion of the Adolescent/Adult Sensory Profile (Brown & Dunn, 2002) identified that he scored much more than most people for low registration, sensory sensitivity and sensation avoiding, and similar to most for sensation seeking. His high neurological threshold for vestibular and proprioceptive information appeared to be resulting in some sensations being perceived as unsafe, in this case the movement of public transport. Jaxon had been highly sensitized to tactile input since the beginning of his psychotic illness and reported that this had not reduced alongside his symptom severity. He described feeling unsafe and found it exceptionally difficult to concentrate if something unexpected touches him. He would be avoidant of situations where unexpected tactile input may occur, such as on public transport, and avoided movement as he did not want to 'set off' uncomfortable extra perceptual tactile experiences. While Jaxon was compliant with his medication, it also had to be considered that his concentration challenges could relate to the negative symptoms of psychosis rather than a sensory processing challenge.

A hypothesis was developed that Jaxon's difficulties with engaging with and completing his college work were due to vestibular hypo-responsivity, tactile hyper-responsivity and decreased opportunity to access regulatory sources of sensory input.

Intervention

Intervention focused on creating a sensory-enhanced routine that promoted Jaxon's ability to engage with external environments. This included identifying sensory strategies to decrease his level of arousal and promoting feelings of safety alongside promoting engagement in activities that provide proprioception to reinforce body awareness and assist with regulating his level of arousal. Jaxon was provided with education in relation to how his sensory processing influences his level of arousal and experience of psychotic symptoms when he feels his safety has been compromised.

CONCLUSION/KEY LEARNING

This chapter considers the evidence in relation to sensory processing changes in psychotic disorders and how sensory-based approaches can be used to support regulation of arousal, reduce feelings of distress and support engagement.

Key points

- Individuals experiencing psychosis have been suggested to show mixed patterns of hyper- and hypo-responsivity as well as difficulties with discrimination of sensory input and impairments in praxis.
- The thalamus is thought to play a key role in these difficulties due to impaired sensory gating.
- These sensory processing differences have been suggested to impact on motor planning, cognitive skills, emotion regulation and functioning.

CHAPTER 3

Borderline Personality Disorder

REBECCA MATSON

Borderline personality disorder (BPD) is a condition commonly associated with difficulties including interpersonal relationships, unstable self-image, poor emotion regulation and impulsivity (APA, 2013). The occupational impact of these difficulties includes decreased motivation and a poor sense of self-efficacy, suggesting a potentially focused role for occupational therapy in supporting establishment of routine in particular (Lee & Harris, 2010). The role of an occupational therapist in evaluating the impact of sensory processing on these areas and using this to inform intervention has received little attention as yet within the literature.

While alterations in sensory processing have been acknowledged within the evidence base, consideration of the impact of these differences and how this should inform approaches to intervention is in relative infancy. Sensory processing differences are not currently considered within diagnostic criteria for BPD but are gaining increasing attention within the literature, with changes in tactile, auditory and interoceptive processing being the most investigated at present. Much of the evidence considered below in relation to alterations in sensory processing comes from outside of occupational therapy literature, which perhaps explains why this is mainly focused on the five more commonly acknowledged senses and lacks the specificity and breadth of sensory integration theory, which guides us to also consider vestibular, interoceptive and proprioceptive processing. The implications of what is known for broader sensory processing will however be considered in view of the neuroscience and sensory integration theory as a whole.

Alterations in sensory processing
Neurological threshold

Individuals with BPD have been found to show altered neurological thresholds that impact on their ability to modulate sensory input; that is, the ability to regulate their response to sensory input in a 'graded and adaptive manner' (Miller et al., 2001, p. 57). A small-scale study using the Adolescent/Adult Sensory Profile (Brown & Dunn, 2002) found a pattern of hyper-responsivity to sensory input to be more prevalent than within both the general population and other diagnostic mental health groups (Brown et al., 2009). Both the categories of sensory sensitivity (where individuals have a lower threshold for sensory input and respond passively to managing this) and sensory avoiding (a lower threshold but actively attempt to manage this) (Dunn, 1997) were heightened for this client group. This pattern of responsivity is highly similar to that identified for those with post-traumatic stress disorder (PTSD), which is perhaps no surprise given that the prevalence of childhood trauma has been suggested to be more than 13 times higher than in the general population and three times higher than other psychiatric populations (Porter et al., 2020). While this is the case, the experience of trauma is not exclusive to this client group and therefore the patterns identified for those who have experienced childhood trauma will be considered in more detail in Chapter 5, PTSD/Trauma.

To understand why these differences may occur and are significant for this client group it is important to consider the underlying neurological processes. Alterations have been found in various areas of the brain integral to sensory processing and integration, including the amygdala, cerebellum, parietal lobe, basal ganglia, thalamus, prefrontal cortex and temporal lobe (Bilek et al., 2019; Khoweiled et al., 2021; Krause-Utz et al., 2021; Malejko et al., 2018; O'Neill et al., 2015). An overview of the role of these areas of the brain in sensory processing and connected processes is provided in Figure 3.1.

One of the primary areas thought to be affected is the thalamus, often referred to as a relay station as the majority of sensory information passes through it and onto other areas of the brain, which has a central role in sensory gating (Bear et al., 2020; Lundy-Eckman, 2013). When sensory gating is ineffective, an individual is likely to be flooded and overwhelmed by too much sensory input, resulting in heightened emotional responses and increased levels of dysregulation. Where sensory gating is excessive for individuals with BPD, it has been suggested to result in difficulties such as dissociative experiences and progressive cognitive dysfunction (Krause-Utz et al., 2021).

However, it should be noted that these two experiences are not necessarily polarized and that individuals with BPD are likely to experience both periods of overwhelm and under-responsivity to sensory input. Bundy and Szklut (2020) suggest the apparently incongruent coinciding of hyper- and hypo-responsivity that can be seen in various populations to be an automatic form of self-protection, rather than a polarized response, where in response to sensory input perceived as a threat, an individual shuts down to prevent being further overwhelmed. This fluctuating or apparently incongruous response can be explained by the hypothalamic–pituitary–adrenal (HPA) axis, a system that mediates our response to stressful experiences or triggers. The HPA axis involves the release of a chain of activating hormones from the hypothalamus, pituitary gland and adrenal gland, which ultimately results in the release of cortisol (Bear et al., 2020). This is a helpful process when we need to respond to a threat but becomes problematic when activated unnecessarily or too easily. Individuals with BPD have been found to experience overactivation of this axis, resulting in a high resting cortisol level and a more easily activated stress response, or 'fight or flight'. As a result, when experiencing an actual threat there is often an apparently blunted or 'freeze' response to perceived stressors (Drews et al., 2019).

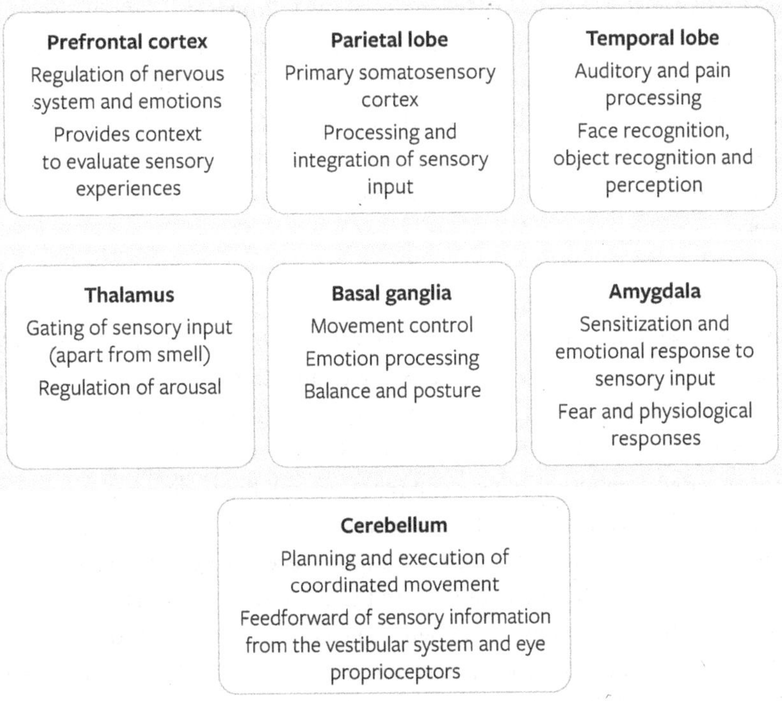

Prefrontal cortex	**Parietal lobe**	**Temporal lobe**
Regulation of nervous system and emotions	Primary somatosensory cortex	Auditory and pain processing
Provides context to evaluate sensory experiences	Processing and integration of sensory input	Face recognition, object recognition and perception

Thalamus	**Basal ganglia**	**Amygdala**
Gating of sensory input (apart from smell)	Movement control	Sensitization and emotional response to sensory input
Regulation of arousal	Emotion processing	
	Balance and posture	Fear and physiological responses

Cerebellum
Planning and execution of coordinated movement
Feedforward of sensory information from the vestibular system and eye proprioceptors

Figure 3.1 Structures of the brain suggested to be affected in borderline personality disorder and their role in relation to sensory processing and connected skills (Bear et al., 2020; Lundy-Eckman, 2013)

Differences in specific sensory systems

TACTILE AND PROPRIOCEPTIVE INPUT

Alterations in somatosensory processing, that is, the processing of tactile and proprioceptive input, have been highlighted in relation to pain perception and intensity of touch (Colle et al., 2020; Löffler et al., 2022; Selby et al., 2022). Löffler et al. (2022) found that tactile experiences were perceived more harshly by individuals with BPD, impacting particularly on what they term 'pleasant touch' experiences such as a hug or affectionate touch on the arm. It is perhaps no surprise with the importance of touch in informing our body awareness that difficulties have also therefore been identified in relation to overall body awareness as well as high levels of dissociation from the body (Schmitz et al., 2021). Touch is also integral to communication, interpersonal relationships and self-soothing (Lane, 2020a), therefore this area of difficulty is perhaps particularly important to consider for individuals with BPD.

AUDITORY PROCESSING

While there has been less discussion of auditory processing in the literature, it has also received attention within studies of BPD (Brown et al., 2009; Rosenthal et al., 2011). Rosenthal et al. (2011) found this to be the sense that evoked the highest level of hyper-responsivity in comparison to healthy controls. However, the measure used within this study, the Self-Perception of Sensory Reactivity, only considered auditory, gustatory, olfactory, visual and tactile processing and not the broader range of sensations acknowledged within sensory integration theory.

INTEROCEPTIVE PROCESSING

Increasing attention is being given to studying alterations in interoceptive processing in this client group due to the connection between interoceptive awareness and emotional regulation and ability to accurately interpret the responses of others (Back & Bertsch, 2020; Löffler et al., 2018). Studies to date have provided conflicting evidence in relation to ability to detect physiological changes such as heartbeat under controlled conditions, with a study by Hart et al. (2013) finding no difference but a more recent study by Flasbeck et al. (2020) concluding that this ability is impaired in this group. There has been suggestion that this ability may depend on factors such as levels of competing external stimuli, with attention becoming directed towards these at the expense of internal signals, due to the increased vigilance often experienced by individuals with BPD (Back & Bertsch, 2020).

Praxis and motor skills

While difficulties in relation to praxis and motor planning are not overtly considered within the literature there is reason to believe occupational therapists should be alert to this possibility and undertake further assessment where relevant. It has been suggested that if an individual spends prolonged periods in a stress state with a chronic activation of the protective system, they then miss important sensory input to inform understanding of and interaction with their environment (Fisher, 1991; Perry, 2009). As a result, they may not receive sufficient information to inform motor planning and praxis (May-Benson, 2017). While this is particularly significant when the sensory systems and motor skills are still developing there is also an apparent impact in adults that has been noted anecdotally in clinical practice. One way in which this is seen is that an individual who is over-responding to sensory input is likely to avoid experiences within that system, limiting potential for receipt of necessary sensory information to inform higher-level skills such as motor planning (Bundy & Szklut, 2020). Difficulties with sensory modulation have also been suggested to potentially mask other sensory processing concerns as well as impacting on ability to make gains within sensory discrimination and praxis (Bundy & Szklut, 2020).

Effective motor planning is dependent on discrimination of tactile, vestibular and proprioceptive input, as well as auditory and visual information (Cermak & May-Benson, 2020). As discussed above, there is some suggestion in the literature of impairments in the ability to discriminate tactile input, particularly in relation to the intensity of the input and pain perception (Löffler et al., 2022). The ability to effectively process and integrate these three sensations is central to the development of body awareness, which Ayres (1972) identified as foundational in informing motor planning. As studies have identified difficulties with both accurate tactile discrimination and body awareness within individuals with BPD there is sufficient reason to consider the possibility of impaired motor planning with this client group.

Impact of sensory processing on functioning

The potential implications of these sensory processing differences for an individual with BPD are significant and are a likely factor in areas identified as diagnostic characteristics such as emotional regulation difficulties, interpersonal relationships, self-image and impulsivity. The relationship between sensory modulation and emotional stability is thought to be a two-way process, with sensitivity to sensory stimuli leading to emotional dysregulation and higher levels of dysregulation leading to a heightened negative response to sensory stimuli (Lane, 2020b); therefore, it would be difficult to ascertain which factor is an initial feature of BPD. Whichever is the initial contributing factor, the sensory sensitivity experienced will have broad implications for maintaining an arousal level that supports positive interactions with others and engagement in meaningful occupations. When an individual is unable to filter out sensations that are not important or relevant at that time, they will struggle to remain present and engaged in a way that supports meaningful engagement in occupations and an adaptive response to their environment.

A sensory lens on self-harm

While self-harm can occur in connection with a range of mental health conditions, it is a coping strategy most commonly connected with borderline personality disorder to the extent that it features in the diagnostic criteria for this condition (APA, 2013). A number of hypotheses have been suggested as to the purpose of or reason for a high level of self-harming behaviours in this population, with the rationale often being connected to emotional regulation and dissociation. One such view is that self-harm serves as a strategy to provide emotional and physical sensations that help regain a connection with the body and the present (Colle et al., 2020). As dissociative experiences lead to an absence of feeling and a sense of distance from reality, the sensations of self-harm can temporarily re-establish this connection.

However, another way to frame the sensory connection of self-harm is as a way to regulate or manage response to sensory stimuli an individual finds difficult to tolerate. Sensory integration theory supports that different sensory inputs can be used to regulate response to triggering sensory inputs (Lane, 2020b), therefore it is possible that self-harm could serve as a way of achieving this. Consider the sensory experiences that are often found to be regulating, particularly deep pressure touch, and linear vestibular and proprioceptive input (Lane, 2020b), and how self-harming behaviours such as head-banging, cutting and insertion of items often provide intense levels of these inputs. While this may be a harmful way of obtaining sensory input, on a neurological level the behaviours may provide sensory input that leads to a sense of release and temporary regulation.

It is also important to consider the evidence for altered pain thresholds within BPD and the likely connection of this with both the method and intensity of self-harm. Individuals with BPD have been suggested to have an overall reduced perception of pain and would require a higher intensity of input in order to fully register and respond to it (Colle et al., 2020). This altered perception of pain is thought to be related to affective and cognitive processing of the stimuli rather than the initial perception of the sensory stimuli or any altered activation of the somatosensory pathways (Malejko et al., 2020). However, in order to achieve heightened awareness an individual may engage in more frequent and more intense methods of self-harm.

Understanding the sensory basis a self-harming behaviour may hold for someone can help both that individual and those working alongside them to develop a greater awareness of the purpose of those actions and potentially decrease the sense of self-blame that often accompanies them. This can also form a starting point to considering sensory inputs that are regulating for that individual prior to considering alternative strategies that may meet the same or a similar need but without causing harm. This is not to say, however, that intervention will be a direct swap of an activity or strategy that provides exactly the same form of sensory input. It may be that other sensory experiences are able to support self-regulation, which thereby reduces the urges to self-harm, but consideration of both approaches is important when working with individuals who self-harm.

Considerations for assessment and intervention

Occupational therapists often first begin working with individuals with BPD when in a highly dysregulated or fluctuating state of arousal, and because of this, the initial focus of sensory-focused work tends to be on reducing the level of risk presentation and identifying 'quick-acting' strategies in the moment rather than achieving longer-term gains. This can make it tempting to rush past the assessment phase to implementing strategies without fully assessing an individual's sensory needs and responses. However, while there may be a need for strategies to provide immediate relief, working solely within this remit would not maximize the full benefits of this approach and could inadvertently lead to strategies which are triggering for that individual. When working with this client group there is often a need for assessment and intervention to run simultaneously and to undergo continuous review in the context of feedback from the client.

As with any client group, a targeted and focused assessment process is needed to best establish needs and priorities for intervention. With difficulties with sensory modulation being most commonly connected with borderline personality disorder, an obvious choice for assessment may be a tool such as the Adolescent/Adult Sensory Profile (Brown & Dunn, 2002), which has a strong focus on sensory modulation in relation to neurological thresholds and behavioural responses. This assessment was used in the study by Brown et al. (2009) and identified sensory processing differences between individuals with BPD and those with other mental health diagnoses. However, when completing an assessment such as this it is important to remember that there is a two-way relationship between sensory modulation and emotional regulation and that the results therefore could be influenced by an individual's current arousal state and may alter once this has decreased.

While difficulties with modulation of sensory input are commonplace in BPD, we need to be careful not to assume this is the full extent of the difficulties experienced by an individual and should be open to the potential need to explore further. Individuals with BPD have been noted to experience a numbing to sensation at times, which could have much broader sensory implications impacting on ability to discriminate sensory input and to successfully integrate sensory input to inform motor skills (Bundy & Szklut, 2020). However, where multiple areas of difficulty have been identified in relation to sensory processing, improving sensory modulation has been highlighted as an important starting point for improving regulation prior to attempting other areas of intervention (Cermak & May-Benson, 2020).

It is perhaps no coincidence that one of the primary approaches currently used with individuals with borderline personality disorder, dialectical behavioural therapy as developed by Linehan (1993), contains sensory-based components within the programme. However, as Moore and McCraith (1998) highlight, the sensory basis of these components does not utilize the full range of sensory inputs, specifically those identified as the 'power senses': deep pressure tactile input, proprioception and vestibular input. Therefore, while sensory-based approaches can work well in tandem with dialectical behaviour therapy, there is a need to ensure focused consideration is given to the regulating impact of these additional sensations.

As discussed briefly above, another consideration for the process is the impact of past experiences on sensory processing. While this will be discussed in more detail in Chapter 5, PTSD/Trauma, it is important to note here that when assessing the impact of sensory processing patterns and planning intervention with this client group, previous trauma should be considered. Experience of trauma-related difficulties such as hyper-vigilance can alter the response to certain sensory experiences, leading to reactions that may appear incongruous (Koomar, 2009). For example, deep pressure touch experiences that may usually be calming to the autonomic nervous system can become triggering due to previous experiences and the psychological connection with this type of touch experience (Koomar, 2009). As a therapist it is important that you explore potential reasons for different sensory responses and also that sensory experiences used in intervention remain within that individual's control.

An important starting point for intervention is providing education in relation to an individual's sensory processing needs and the impact of this on their self-regulation and functioning. A significant benefit of sensory modulation approaches for this client group is the ability to be self-led and the resultant sense of control this returns to that individual (Matson et al., 2021). While there are often benefits to involvement of others, such as staff, workers or family members, in the early days of learning to use strategies while self-awareness is building, to ensure longevity of strategy use there is a need for individuals to have a greater understanding not only of their sensory processing patterns but also of the rationale for why they may find specific sensory strategies effective. This is not only likely to support longer-term use but also may enable that individual to identify further strategies that work on a similar basis and maximize levels of independence in this area.

Finally, there is a need to consider the risk of self-harm and whether plans for intervention may increase this risk in any way. Identifying a potential risk does not automatically mean a planned activity or strategy cannot go ahead but may mean additional measures need to be in place. As occupational therapists we have a duty to manage risk where possible and to avoid putting our clients at undue risk (Royal College of Occupational Therapists (RCOT), 2021), and this needs to form a central part of our considerations for intervention. However, when individuals value a strategy, risk of self-harm with the items provided often decreases significantly and therapeutic risk-taking is enabled.

Strategies and approaches

While not all individuals with BPD will be identified as having clinically significant differences in sensory processing, all may benefit from the use of sensory-based strategies to support self-regulation. There does not have to be a particular difficulty with sensory processing in order to benefit from the therapeutic use of certain inputs, just as we all use different sensory experiences to alter our arousal state on a day-to-day basis.

Sensory support plans or safety plans

Safety plans are not an intervention unique to sensory intervention and are often used when working with individuals who are at high risk of self-harm behaviours to help provide direction or prompts towards alternative strategies to support them when in distress (O'Sullivan & Fitzgibbon, 2018). Depending on both individual preference and level of insight, this plan may be developed to be used by the person themselves or by those around them, such as staff or carers, to help engage that person in strategies that are likely to support de-escalation.

The focus of a sensory support or safety plan is to identify both the sensory experiences that are helpful alongside the times or situations when they should be used and the intended effect. These plans tend to be most effective when they include both 'in the moment' reactive strategies as well as proactive strategies to improve overall levels of regulation. Individuals often struggle to identify the more proactive strategies when in a state of high dysregulation, therefore it may be necessary to start within introducing reactive strategies initially and then further develop the plan. While a more comprehensive list of sensory-based strategies is provided in Chapter 10, Sensory Strategies, as well as ideas of how to incorporate these into a focused plan, below are ideas of strategies in relation to three common priority areas of intervention for individuals with BPD: reactive strategies, proactive strategies and body awareness strategies.

Reactive strategies

Reactive strategies are designed to support de-escalation of arousal levels and therefore are most effective when low demand and focused on providing short sharp bursts of sensory input. Below are some examples in relation to a range of sensory inputs:

- Pushing hard against a gym ball. This primarily provides proprioceptive input and can be done either directly against a wall or another person.
- Putting aromatherapy oils on a tissue or piece of material.
    - Smells are highly effective in grounding, but due to a strong emotional connection these should be trialled first while in a lower arousal state to identify if the impact is positive.
- Sucking on a sour sweet or strong mint or biting into a lemon can provide alerting input that can support grounding and divert attention from distressing thoughts.
- Using spiky massage balls provides deeper tactile input where the individual can alter the intensity.
- Bouncing rhythmically on a gym ball. It is important that this is linear and gentle to prevent it from increasing arousal levels.

Proactive strategies

Using proactive strategies will help prevent an increase in arousal levels and support engagement with others and in meaningful occupations. Below are examples of activities and strategies that can help to incorporate regulating input into an individual's day.

- Timetabling of movement-based activities that provide proprioceptive input into the day.
- Categorizing music into that which is triggering and that which helps to positively alter mood.
- Using 'fidget tools' such as tangle fidgets or stress balls can help provide small amounts of regulating input when engaged in an activity.
- Progressive muscle relaxation. While not an activity developed within sensory integration practice it provides high amounts of regulating proprioceptive input.
- Baking or cooking activities that involve actions such as kneading.
- Using a white noise app or machine, or preferred music through in-ear headphones, to block out other sounds where auditory sensitivity is a concern.
- Using a vibration cushion or pad.
    - For some individuals who find deep pressure input triggering this can be easier to tolerate; however, it should be trialled initially when in a lower state of arousal.
- Exercising on gym machines on high resistance to increase proprioceptive input.
- Incorporating calming sensory inputs into a personal care routine, for example using a vibration toothbrush, scented products containing aromas identified as calming for that individual, or using a loofah or body puff to provide deeper tactile input.

Activities to improve body awareness

As discussed above, decreased body awareness has been identified in individuals with BPD. Our body awareness not only provides a physical awareness but also connects with feelings of safety and improved regulation (Cermak & May-Benson, 2020; Schmitz et al., 2021). Therefore, improving connection with the body could have a significant impact for an individual with BPD. The most effective way to increase body awareness is through providing increased input from the 'power senses' of proprioception, vestibular input and tactile input, specifically deep pressure touch and vibration (Bundy & Szklut, 2020). Caution should be taken with the tactile strategies particularly, and if an individual is reluctant to try a certain strategy trust their response, as this may be a safety reaction.

- Add in weight to everyday activities, such as walking to the shop, through use of ankle or wrist weights or items such as a weighted backpack.
- Swimming is a great activity for providing all three of these inputs at the same time, thereby supporting improved overall integration.
- Body-weight exercises such as holding a plank or press-ups.
- Yoga poses are another activity that is great for providing input through all three sensory systems. To increase proprioceptive input through heightened muscle stretch try introducing the use of yoga blocks.
- Weightlifting activities provide high levels of muscle input that support development of body scheme.
- Using an electric toothbrush can provide regulating tactile input through vibration.
- Rocking chair or swings to provide linear vestibular input.
- Compression garments provide deep pressure touch input. Similar input can be obtained through Lycra clothing or tight-fitting jeans.
- High resistance stress balls such as hand exercisers. These help provide increased levels of muscle tension but are lower demand than body-weight exercises.
- Weighted modalities such as a weighted blanket or weighted shawl – introduce cautiously where there is a history of trauma as this sensation can be dysregulating for some.
- Massage tools, like spiky massage balls, help provide deep pressure input that is in the control of the individual themselves where they can choose to alter the intensity or location of the input.
    - Vibrating massage tools are an alternative that provides a different form of touch input that some find easier to tolerate.

CASE STUDY – Aoife
Background
Aoife, a 19-year-old with a diagnosis of borderline personality disorder, was residing in an inpatient mental health service following a period of increased incidents of self-harm, a number of which required treatment at hospital. Aoife described her self-harm urges as occurring following a build-up of tension in her body which she needed to release. Aoife could rapidly shift into a state of dysregulation and was not always aware of what had triggered this. Aoife found the level of sensory stimulation on the ward difficult to tolerate, particularly the noises and others unexpectedly touching her, and as a result had been spending increased periods of time in her room to

manage this. Aoife was highly creative and enjoyed spending time engaging in activities such as crochet and painting. Aoife had an aim to go to college following discharge to complete an art course, but was worried about how she would manage the college environment.

Assessment and formulation of difficulties

Aoife completed an Adolescent/Adult Sensory Profile (Brown & Dunn, 2002), which identified heightened levels of avoidance in relation to tactile, vestibular and auditory input. Aoife's scores also suggested increased levels of low registration to these inputs; however, in discussion with her occupational therapist, Aoife identified that this reflected periods of dissociation where she found herself becoming 'numb' and often followed times where she had become overwhelmed. Aoife's self-harm often involved methods that provided deep pressure input such as cutting and inserting items into wounds.

Intervention

Aoife began by working with her occupational therapist to identify strategies that would help 'in the moment' when she felt the sense of tension beginning to build and provide her with an alternative option. Initially wearing a Lycra sleeve proved effective but Aoife reported finding herself tightening it on her arm to increase the pressure to the extent that it would inhibit the blood flow. The next option trialled was a hand exerciser which allowed Aoife to gain tension in her arm and receive proprioceptive input. This proved more effective as Aoife could alter the level of tension, and also reduced the risk of harming herself when using the strategy. Aoife was also shown a range of body-tensing exercises but found the visual cue of the exerciser helped her to make that choice in the moment.

Focus then moved to strategies to improve overall levels of regulation and decrease responsivity to sensory triggers from the environment, examples of which follow. Aoife found lavender to be a calming scent for her as it was connected with positive memories, and so chose to create a lavender spray that she could spray around her room but also take with her in her bag when she went out. Aoife tried using white noise but found this could irritate her at times and so changed to instead using her preferred music on headphones as a strategy for coping with problematic noises. She created a playlist with songs that helped her to feel calmer in response to different emotions and identified those that she shouldn't listen to when struggling to regulate as they could make her become more agitated. Aoife enjoyed baking, therefore opportunities for proprioception to improve overall regulation were added into her meal preparation routine where possible and she began making meals such as homemade pizza where she would need to work the dough.

CONCLUSION/KEY LEARNING

This chapter considers the evidence in relation to sensory processing changes in borderline personality disorder, including the potential connection of this to traumatic experiences. Awareness of the impact of sensory processing can enable a reframing of some of the difficulties experienced in relation to emotion regulation, functioning and social engagement.

Key points

- Individuals with a diagnosis of BPD have been suggested to show primarily heightened sensory responsivity but with periods of 'shutdown' and apparent decreased responsivity.
- The HPA axis is thought to play a key role in this dysregulation and connected difficulties.
- A mixture of reactive (in the moment) and proactive strategies is likely to be most beneficial in grounding and supporting regulation of arousal.

CHAPTER 4

Eating Disorders

REBECCA MATSON

Occupational therapists often have an active role in working with individuals with an eating disorder, including supporting the completion of occupations that have become problematic in the context of an eating disorder; re-establishing engagement in a broader range of occupations that have declined; and establishing an identity outside of the eating disorder (Sørlie et al., 2020). The role of an occupational therapist in evaluating the impact of sensory processing on the experience of an eating disorder and in considering these factors in the treatment process has started to receive attention within the literature, but most research into how sensory processing may be altered is outside of occupational therapy literature.

Eating disorders have been described as a 'severe and persistent disturbance in eating behaviours and associated distressing thoughts and emotions' (APA, 2023). The DSM-5 (APA, 2013) considers a number of eating disorders, but within this chapter focus will be given to three of the most commonly identified, anorexia nervosa, bulimia nervosa and binge eating disorder, as these three have received the greatest consideration in relation to sensory processing within the literature to date. Criteria used to distinguish these three disorders include:

- Anorexia nervosa: Persistent restricted food intake leading to significant reduction in weight below the expected BMI. Often features an extreme fear of weight gain and can include behaviours intended to control weight such as excessive exercise and laxative use.
- Bulimia nervosa: Repeated periods of binging on food followed by activities intended to counteract weight gain such as purging through vomiting, excessive exercise or use of laxatives.
- Binge eating disorder: Involves repeated periods of binging on high quantities of food often until uncomfortably full. May also include eating

much quicker and consuming large amounts of food when not hungry. (APA, 2013; Brockmeyer et al., 2018)

Avoidant/restrictive food intake disorder (ARFID) has been acknowledged as a specific eating disorder since 2013 (APA, 2013) but with a different presentation to other eating disorders in that concerns about weight or body shape are not a feature of this condition. One of the potential presentations with ARFID entails a sensory sensitivity that leads to avoidance of foods due to factors such as texture, taste or appearance (Thomas et al., 2017). While ARFID will not be considered in any detail in this chapter, there are considerations discussed below that are likely to have relevance when working with this client group such as those relating to low body weight which, while not a preoccupation in ARFID, will have an impact that needs to be considered.

Alterations in sensory processing
Neurological threshold

Heightened levels of sensory sensitivity, and therefore a lower neurological threshold, have been suggested in individuals with anorexia nervosa (AN), through comparisons to both those with bulimia nervosa (BN) and the general population, suggesting that this may be a commonly experienced trait (Bell et al., 2017; Galiana-Simal et al., 2017). While a connection of this sensitivity with the impact of malnutrition resulting from food restriction has been hypothesized, the level of difference experienced is thought to be beyond the impact of this, suggesting malnutrition is not the sole cause (Galiana-Simal et al., 2017). However, this finding is not consistent across the literature, with some studies suggesting a different pattern of reduced responsivity in those with AN and a heightened responsivity in those experiencing BN (Bell et al., 2017).

One theory here is that sensory responsivity may vary depending on factors such as weight restoration, with sensory perception improving as weight increases, and therefore is more strongly connected with illness severity rather than the specific condition (Gaudio et al., 2014). However, other studies have found that this heightened sensitivity persists regardless of variations in weight and malnutrition, and that this instead varies according to the specific sense being considered (Brand-Gothelf et al., 2016). Brand-Gothelf et al. (2016) found levels of sensory sensitivity to be higher in individuals following a restoration in weight, suggesting that there is a dulling in sensory responsivity experienced during a severe episode of an eating disorder.

One distinction suggested when considering level of responsivity to sensory stimuli is whether the input is interoceptive or exteroceptive; an individual with an eating disorder may have difficulty balancing these two factors (Cobbaert et al., 2024; Herbert, 2020). Herbert (2020) suggests this results from the high perceived threat level from internal stimuli leading to an individual 'shutting down', or reduction of the attention given to these cues, and therefore the individual experiences lower levels of interoceptive input. These interoceptive difficulties have been identified as increasing the lower the BMI is, and as being experienced to a greater level in those with AN and BN in comparison to individuals with binge eating disorder (BED) (Jenkinson et al., 2018). The level of interoceptive difficulties experienced has been found to be most heightened in BN (Cobbaert et al., 2024).

In a study using the Adolescent/Adult Sensory Profile (Brown & Dunn, 2002), Saure et al. (2022) analysed the sensory processing patterns of individuals with AN, including evaluation of differences according to the specific subtype, restrictive (AN-R) or binge purge type (AN-BP). They found significant differences for individuals with AN of both types in relation to all domains (low registration, sensory seeking, sensory sensitivity and sensory avoiding) in comparison with healthy controls. Those with AN-R were found to show lower levels of sensation seeking but higher levels of sensory sensitivity and sensory avoiding, whereas those with AN-BP showed higher levels of low registration, sensory sensitivity and sensory avoiding. Both groups showed a significantly higher level of hyper-responsivity in comparison with the control group (Saure et al., 2022). This is similar to the findings of Brand-Gothelf et al. (2016) of heightened sensitivity in those with AN-R that correlated with severity of the eating disorder symptoms. Individuals with BN, however, showed higher levels of sensory hypo-responsivity than those with AN-R.

These alterations in sensory responsivity have been connected with increased dysregulation of the hypothalamic–pituitary–adrenal (HPA) axis and higher levels of emotion dysregulation in individuals with AN in particular (Sim & Peterson, 2021). A chronic overactivation of the hypothalamic–pituitary–adrenal axis has been suggested in AN that, while thought to initially occur in connection with restriction of dietary intake, does not necessarily return to normal functioning following recovery (Puckett et al., 2021). This results in an overactivation of the sympathetic nervous system and therefore heightened cortisol levels and an altered threat response (Munro et al., 2016). Prolonged periods of overactivation within this axis tend to result in fluctuating emotion regulation and responsivity to sensory input. This may therefore help to explain the differing patterns of sensory responsivity seen within anorexia nervosa in particular. Increased activation has also been noted in the insula and cingulate, areas that have been connected with altered sensitivity to sensory input in eating disorders (Acevedo et al., 2021; Sim & Peterson, 2021). Figure 4.1 illustrates this pattern of reactivity.

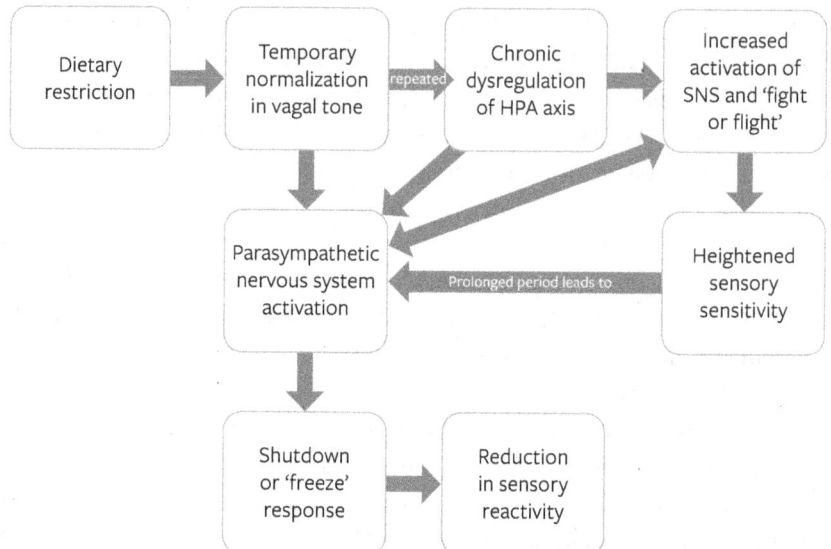

Figure 4.1 Fluctuating responsivity to sensory input in anorexia nervosa (based on Sim & Peterson, 2021)

Whether alterations in sensory processing precede the onset of an eating disorder or occur as a result of it is not known. Overall, however, the presence of atypical sensory processing has been connected with increased severity of eating disorder symptoms and higher levels of self-disgust (Bell et al., 2017; Brand-Gothelf et al., 2016; Saure et al., 2022). Saure et al. (2022) suggest that individuals with AN and sensory processing differences are likely to experience increased challenges in the treatment process and require consideration of alternative interventions to those traditionally utilized, which is where sensory-based interventions should be considered.

Differences in specific sensory systems

Individuals with eating disorders have been found to experience altered sensory processing in relation to interoception and tactile, proprioceptive, visual and gustatory input, with certain areas being more prevalent depending on the nature of the eating disorder. Response to gustatory input has received surprisingly little attention but there is some suggestion of alterations in perception of bitter, sweet and acidic tastes. However, whether this is hyper-responsivity or hypo-responsivity varies between studies (Brand-Gothelf et al., 2016; Harrison et al., 2019).

INTEROCEPTIVE PROCESSING

The area that has received the most attention is interoceptive awareness with alterations being found in both AN and BN to a much greater extent than those with a diagnosis of binge eating disorder (BED) and greater impairment correlating with lower BMI (Brown et al., 2017; Cobbaert et al., 2024; Jenkinson et al., 2018). Difficulties in this area have been suggested to be most apparent in those with BN (Jenkinson et al., 2018). This has been found to correlate with awareness of being hungry and being full, but also with perception of heartbeat (Herbert, 2020; Yamamotova et al., 2017), and is thought to relate to a threat response resulting in an increase or decrease in the level of responsivity to these sensations as a form of self-protection (Herbert, 2020). Another hypothesis is that increased attention is often directed towards external sensory stimuli, that is, visual input and perception of the body, which diverts awareness away from internal stimuli (Eshkevari et al., 2014).

TACTILE INPUT

Differences in people with an eating disorder have been found that relate to both internal and external perception of tactile stimuli. This area of difficulty has been specifically connected with those with AN, with alterations being found in relation to both modulation and discrimination of tactile input (Bell et al., 2017; Brand-Gothelf et al., 2016; Gaudio et al., 2014; Sim & Peterson, 2021). Individuals with AN demonstrate hyper-responsivity to external tactile input but a decreased awareness of pain (Bell et al., 2017; Brand-Gothelf et al., 2016; Sim & Peterson, 2021). Gaudio et al. (2014) highlight decreased levels of sensory perception for individuals with AN, impacting on both tactile and proprioceptive awareness, and connect this with alterations in the parietal lobe. They highlight this as a significant factor in reduced body awareness for those with AN. Tactile and proprioceptive input are integral in development of our internal body map (Bundy & Lane, 2020), therefore reduced perception of both of these inputs could be highly significant for an individual with an eating disorder, resulting in an overall disconnection with the body and inability to challenge their altered perception of factors such as weight and body shape.

VISUAL INPUT

Increased sensitivity to visual input is also an area highlighted specifically in relation to AN, with the suggestion that this leads to decreased attention to other sensory information (Eshkevari et al., 2014). There has also been suggestion of difficulties integrating visual information with other sensory inputs, such as proprioception and tactile input, further enhancing inaccuracies in body awareness (Gaudio et al., 2014; Yamamotova et al., 2017). Riva and Dakanalis (2018), however, suggest a broader difficulty relating to multi-sensory integration overall and an impact on ability to both accurately interpret interoceptive signals and accurately evaluate body scheme.

Impact of sensory processing on functioning

While the exact impact of these difficulties on functioning is not known, there is the potential for them to be factors in a number of areas of concern connected with occupational functioning such as eating, shopping, dressing and social functioning. There is a temptation to view all behaviours or difficulties in the context of eating disorder pathology without considering the impact of sensory processing on areas such as avoidance of specific foods, seeking of certain types of movement and a preference for certain clothing types. For occupational therapists working in this area, it is important that these aspects are evaluated to help provide targeted and supportive intervention (Saure et al., 2022).

Difficulties in tolerating particular foods, for example, could be the result of variation in textures, the temperature of food or the taste or smell of certain items rather than the calorie intake connected with them. Cobbaert et al. (2024) identified in their systematic review a heightened sensitivity to taste being particularly prevalent in AN and suggest that approaches to intervention need to consider this and aim to provide increased predictability in food and more bland tastes in order to support increased dietary intake. Programmes designed to support eating disorder recovery often require following a highly prescribed dietary intake initially designed to aid weight restoration, but it is important that the presence of such difficulties is considered if this process is to be successful and support establishment of longer-term eating habits. If sensory difficulties in this area are not acknowledged, then as that individual attempts to move away from a highly prescribed diet this could result in unexpected barriers, particularly when attempting to engage in social eating activities where the food may be less predictable and the experience altered by the smells of other people's food or different levels of flavourings used within a meal. Similarly, a preference for loose-fitting clothing is often thought to be a desire to hide body shape but could in fact relate to a dislike of the tactile sensation of tight-fitting clothing.

A sensory lens on exercise and movement

One area of concern that is often viewed from the lens of eating disorder symptomology is engagement in high levels of exercise or a persistent seeking of movement. Both may be features of an eating disorder, with the primary intention to propagate weight loss, but it is important to consider whether this is the intended purpose for a specific individual or whether this is a way of meeting sensory needs. In the early stages of eating disorder treatment there is often a focus on reducing levels of movement, but if an individual has a need for high levels of proprioception and vestibular input to feel regulated then this could be a potential barrier in the recovery process.

An individual may seek movement for a range of reasons, and one of these could be for the sensory benefits and connected regulation. Proprioceptive input in particular supports regulation of responsivity to other sensory inputs and emotion regulation, and informs increased body awareness, all of which are areas of concern in eating disorders (Blanche & Schaaf, 2001). Similarly, while vestibular input can perhaps be more easily received through relatively passive activities, such as using a rocking chair, this is not likely to achieve the same regulating benefits as when received in purposeful movement.

That is not to say that it may not be necessary to encourage a reduction in the intensity or amount of physical exercise in order to support physical recovery, and there are points when this becomes very much a necessity to preserve life; it can even be necessary to reduce movement by a significant level for a period of time. Where this is necessary it is important to evaluate the purpose of such activities for an individual, and if there are sensory benefits consider how these can be met in other ways, either temporarily or in the longer term. Identifying the purpose of physically active activities is an important part of the role of an occupational therapist both in supporting that individual in achieving a regulated state and establishing their occupational identity through the recovery process.

Considerations for assessment and intervention

Occupational therapists are generally acknowledged as having a key role in the treatment of eating disorders due to the impact on activities of daily living as well as occupational identity (Dark & Carter, 2020; Lawrence & Mcauley, 2023). There is often a need for focused intervention in relation to meal preparation, food shopping, eating, restoration of engagement in a variety of occupations that may have been narrowed due to a fixation on food, and development of coping skills (Sørlie et al., 2020). Sensory processing may be a key factor in many of these activities and also an important consideration in establishing a level of regulation that enables engagement in valued activities and relationships with others.

Identification of sensory processing patterns may support necessary dietary considerations, in view of factors such as aversion to certain textures or tastes and planning of therapeutic activities, and also support an increase in self-regulation. Completion of a sensory assessment may provide greater insight both to the person themselves but also to the team working with them that can inform the overall recovery process. Awareness of such factors could be integral in the recovery process to support establishing of habits that are sustainable and reduce potential barriers within the process. This could also be highly empowering for that individual in providing a rationale for some of the areas of difficulty experienced.

The primary areas of difficulty identified within the literature tend to relate to sensory modulation, and therefore the Adolescent/Adult Sensory Profile (AASP) (Brown & Dunn, 2002) may be a suitable choice; however, this does not currently capture interoceptive awareness, which is a central area of concern for this client group. A connected form is in development, the Sensory Profile Interoception (SPI) scale (Brown & Dunn, 2023), which assesses interoception in the context of participation and has been found to have high construct validity, internal consistency and concurrent validity (Brown & Dunn, 2023; Dunn et al., 2022). This is likely to be a tool of value when working with this client group.

One difficulty in the assessment process, however, is that there are a number of questions on an assessment such as the AASP which may not measure the factor intended and could be reflective of eating disorder symptomology or its impact, rather than sensory processing. Therefore, when completing any form of sensory assessment, it is important to obtain qualitative data to support the process of interpretation. For example, the experience of dizziness may be influenced by insufficient dietary intake rather than alterations in vestibular processing. The same caution may be needed in relation to questions screening for a need to move, which may be reflective of sensory processing needs or an intention to burn calories, and questions relating to the avoidance of certain food types or tastes.

A thorough assessment is an important starting point, but one of the main barriers to sensory-based interventions with eating disorders is the difficulty of providing certain sensory inputs that may have been identified as necessary or beneficial for an individual. When an individual is experiencing high levels of dysregulation, as can often be the case with eating disorders, the most effective sensory inputs tend to be proprioception, deep pressure touch and linear vestibular input (Bundy & Szklut, 2020). All of these can present increased challenges when working with individuals with an eating disorder due to the demands they place on the body. Proprioceptive input is particularly problematic with a low BMI as it depends on high levels of active resistance and muscle tension, which are potentially unsafe when this is the case. Common areas of concern when working with individuals low in weight include muscle and bone density and cardiac irregularities, all of which are potential risk factors when engaging in physically strenuous activities (Quesnel et al., 2023). The Safe Exercise at Every Stage (SEES) guidance document (Dobinson et al., 2019) provides evidence-based information to support consideration of relevant factors and inform your clinical reasoning and may be of use when attempting to identify activities that could safely support provision of desired sensory inputs.

Where this is a concern alternatives may need to be considered to support an individual to receive regulating sensory inputs while avoiding putting them at increased risk. One alternative is to support engagement in activities that provide muscle stretch rather than tension through assuming certain positions, such as yoga postures, rather than high levels of exertion. Another option is considering the use of deep pressure touch and vibration, which also support increased regulation but in a more passive manner, and in a similar way vestibular input that requires lower exertion. Examples of activities that do this are provided in the section below.

Caution will need to be taken with all activities and it will be important to consult your multi-disciplinary team, particularly if working with a low BMI, to support engagement in activity that considers calorie intake and physical observations where needed.

Strategies and approaches

Regardless of whether an individual with an eating disorder has identified differences in sensory processing, there are likely to be benefits in using sensory-based strategies to support their overall self-regulation. Strategies discussed below include those that may support general regulation, those that could help reduce sensory sensitivity and improve body awareness, and strategies to develop interoception. We all have our own sensory responses, and therefore identifying the most effective strategies to support an individual's self-regulation is likely to take trial and error. This is best guided by the use of a sensory checklist to help identify sensory inputs likely to be most beneficial to that individual. Further guidance on strategy ideas and incorporating these into a focused plan is included in Chapter 10, Sensory Strategies, with the guidance below providing more client-group-specific ideas.

Strategies to support regulation

- Yoga is perhaps one of the best activities for providing regulating inputs while placing a lower demand on the body.
    - Levels of proprioceptive input can be increased through muscle stretch, which can be enhanced further through using yoga blocks.
    - To provide vestibular input consider poses that encourage inversion of the head.

- Using a vibration cushion can provide regulating input that travels along the same pathways as deep pressure touch input and therefore tends to be calming.

- Using massage tools supports provision of deep pressure touch input but in a way that can be controlled by the individual, therefore may be a good place to start if an individual has been identified as experiencing tactile sensitivity.
    - Caution is needed where skin integrity may be reduced.

- Using an electric toothbrush is another way to provide deep pressure touch but can also help decrease tactile sensitivity in the mouth.

- Smelling aromatherapy oils. It may take trial and error to identify a smell that is beneficial for each individual, but this can be an effective way to support regulation and also could be used to counter the smells of problematic foods.

- Listening to music. Supporting an individual to identify calming music can be helpful for situations they find triggering such as meal times.

- Using a weighted blanket provides deep pressure touch.
    - Caution needs to be taken to follow guidelines in relation to proportionate weight and potential risk factors. RCOT (2023) recommend caution where skin integrity or regulation of temperature is an issue and that the blanket should not exceed more than 10 per cent of body weight. Due to the potential for fluctuations in body weight

with this client group this would need to be closely reviewed and monitored.

- Using a weighted shawl could provide similar input to a blanket but with less intensity; alternatively a rice- or bead-filled cushion could be used, with the weight adjusted as needed.

- Incorporating calming sensory inputs into meal preparation through activities such as kneading bread or mixing ingredients will create small amounts of proprioceptive input.

- Gardening activities will need to be considered in view of factors such as weight. The intensity of inputs can be effectively altered and full-body activities such as digging can be replaced with potting of plants or using a trowel in a flower bed.

- Drinking through a straw provides regulating oral-motor input that could be used at meal times to support regulation around eating.

Strategies to support body awareness

Body awareness is most effectively increased through provision of proprioceptive, vestibular and tactile input, all of which can contain challenges when working with this client group. Below are some ideas for how these inputs can be provided to varying extents depending on the current level of caution needed:

- Swimming provides all three of these sensory inputs in an integrated way but with the level of demand on joints reduced due to the movement being in water.

- Yoga poses – poses that involve greater muscle stretch will be most effective in developing body awareness but those that require focus on breathing can also be helpful in this respect.

- Wearing body socks/dance socks. These can be called different things depending on the supplier but are usually made of a Lycra material that helps to provide opportunities for low levels of resistance and touch input.

- Massage tools used on different parts of the body provide deep pressure touch input that can increase awareness of the body.

- Squeezing items such as Theraputty or hand exercises provides an opportunity for muscle tension that is controlled by the individual.

- Progressive muscle relaxation. Various versions of this are available both pre-recorded and in the form of scripts. The tension of different body parts during these exercises helps build awareness of body scheme through proprioceptive input.

Strategies for development of interoception

Awareness of how to increase interoceptive abilities in relation to sensations is a developing area of knowledge but there are resources and programmes available to support this. There tend to be two main factors in the approach to increasing interoceptive awareness:

- Putting in place adaptive strategies or supports: These tend to be used in the early stages while interoception is building. This could be strategies such as timers to remind someone when to eat or use the toilet. Scheduling of meals and snacks is a common part of eating disorder intervention, therefore nothing additional may be needed in this area. Consideration may also need to be given to portion sizes where an individual struggles with feelings of fullness to support a gradual increase in dietary intake and ability to tolerate these feelings (Cobbaert & Rose, 2023). Use of calming strategies that involve other sensory inputs, such as those discussed above, may be beneficial prior to meal times to increase overall regulation in preparation for this challenge.

- Activities designed to build awareness of interoception: Examples could include body scan exercises, mindfulness exercises, breathing exercises and progressive muscle relaxation. All of these help to increase focus on internal sensations. These may need to be used cautiously during the early stages of recovery when increasing this focus could be triggering, and therefore consultation with other members of the multi-disciplinary team where available would be advisable. Programmes such as the Interoception Curriculum (Mahler, 2019), while designed for use with children, may also contain useful ideas and exercises to support with this process when working with adults.

CASE STUDY – Joanne
Background
Joanne, a 29-year-old woman with a diagnosis of anorexia nervosa, was under the care of the community eating disorder service. Joanne had a BMI of 14 following a recent inpatient admission to stabilize her physical health and support increased dietary intake. Joanne had been known to exercise to excessive levels, but also reported having enjoyed sports as a teenager and that exercise benefited her wellbeing prior to development of her eating disorder. Joanne reported that when unable to exercise she would become increasingly agitated and withdrawn. Joanne also became overwhelmed in supermarkets by the bright lighting and noise or other shoppers, and this increased her reluctance to shop for food, which was already an anxiety-provoking activity for her.

Assessment and formulation of difficulties
Completion of an Adolescent/Adult Sensory Profile (Brown & Dunn, 2002) with Joanne identified heightened levels of sensitivity and avoidance, low registration in relation to auditory, visual and touch input, and seeking of movement input. Joanne appeared to be experiencing fluctuating responsivity suggestive of difficulties with modulating auditory, visual and touch input, which were likely to be impacting on her ability to access the supermarket. However, as heightened arousal levels increase an individual's responsivity to sensory input, her apparent elevated anxiety levels when accessing the supermarket, which could also be due to the food-related nature of the activity, may also have been leading to this heightened responsivity to problematic sensory inputs. Joanne's seeking of movement activities was considered to be a potential way of regulating her responsivity to these other sensory inputs.

Intervention
Joanne had a relatively low BMI and therefore caution was needed in the use of movement-based strategies due to the potential for over-exertion and reduction in muscle and bone density. There was also a need to balance dietary intake with level of exercise to ensure she had sufficient energy to engage in any identified activities and that the activities did not lead to further weight loss. The therapist used the SEES guidelines to help consider what movement activities may be advisable, identifying yoga as a suitable movement-based activity but keeping to gentle exercises initially for a maximum of 30 minutes. As Joanne achieved further weight restoration this was

reviewed and increased to poses that involved greater stretch to maximize the proprioceptive input she received from this.

To help with managing the level of stimulation when accessing the supermarket Joanne began listening to music she found calming on headphones. Joanne began using a weighted blanket for a short period prior to leaving home to reduce her arousal levels and help her to feel calmer. Joanne also took a hand exerciser with her when shopping that she kept in her pocket to allow her to squeeze it when she felt herself becoming overwhelmed within the shop. This helped her to pause and refocus when in the shop and complete her shopping without becoming overwhelmed.

CONCLUSION/KEY LEARNING

This chapter considers the evidence in relation to sensory processing changes in eating disorders and how this might vary between anorexia, bulimia and binge eating disorder. Understanding more about these underlying difficulties can inform a more individualized approach to intervention in view of sensory preferences.

Key points

- Sensory reactivity in eating disorders has been suggested to be impacted by variations in weight and conflicts between interoceptive and exteroceptive sensory signals.
- Considering eating and activity preferences in view of sensory responses may support an individualized formulation of difficulties.
- Sensory-based approaches can support improved regulation and interoceptive awareness.

CHAPTER 5

PTSD/Trauma

REBECCA MATSON

Post-traumatic stress disorder (PTSD) can occur following experiencing or being witness to a traumatic event. Traumatic experiences encompass a range of life events and factors which may include abuse, violence, neglect, war and/or emotional harm (APA, 2013). PTSD is characterized by repeatedly re-experiencing the event, avoidance behaviours, hyper-vigilance and heightened arousal levels (APA, 2013). The impact of traumatic experiences on sensory processing has been acknowledged both within the field of occupational therapy and the broader fields of mental health and neuroscience (Harrichan et al., 2021; Joseph et al., 2021). This impact is particularly evident in complex trauma, which relates to prolonged experiences such as ongoing abuse or neglect, rather than singular incidents. Such trauma alters both the developmental process and the formation of healthy attachments (Van der Kolk, 2005, 2015).

Trauma has been suggested to interrupt the foundational process of sensory integration itself, particularly when it occurs at an early age, altering the development of neural connections and impacting both cognitive development and sensory processing (Holland & May-Benson, 2014; Matson et al., 2024; Van der Kolk, 2005). While the literature regarding trauma and sensory processing primarily relates to children, the difficulties identified are likely to continue into adulthood if intervention is not received as a child. As a result, trauma has the potential to affect an individual's roles and occupations throughout their life (Champagne & Pfeiffer, 2020). Therefore, literature relating to both life stages is included within this chapter.

Experience of early trauma has been connected with various mental health conditions, including post-traumatic stress disorder (PTSD), borderline personality disorder (BPD), psychosis, anxiety and depression (Karaca Dinç et al., 2021; McGreevy & Bolland, 2020), leading to a focus within mental health services on trauma-informed care. Therefore, the evidence and ideas presented within this chapter are likely to be of relevance in supporting this trauma-informed approach whatever your client group.

Alterations in sensory processing
Neurological threshold

Differing views exist on the neurological threshold of individuals who have experienced trauma, with some sources suggesting a fluctuating response to sensory input in which the same individuals demonstrate both hyper-responsivity and hypo-responsivity at differing times, and others suggesting the pattern of responsivity relates to specific factors in the experience of trauma. Engel-Yeger et al. (2013) found that when assessed using the Adolescent/Adult Sensory Profile (Brown & Dunn, 2002), adults with PTSD showed higher levels of both hyper-responsivity and hypo-responsivity to sensory input, which initially may appear contradictory. However, they postulated that the apparent hypo-responsivity was an extension of the continuum of hyper-responsivity, where individuals with PTSD become so overwhelmed by sensory input that they present with periods of 'shutdown' as a protective automatic response to manage this. In this state of shutdown individuals tend to present as numb, immobilized and unresponsive to those around them, and to sensory input (Ogden, 2021), and therefore present as if hypo-responsive. This fluctuating pattern has been echoed in a study completed with individuals with unipolar and bipolar depression who had experienced childhood trauma (Serafini et al., 2016), and studies relating to traumatized children (Joseph et al., 2022).

Kearney and Lanius (2022) suggest another explanation, relating the pattern seen to the presence or absence of dissociative symptoms. In their view hypo-responsivity is the result of an individual experiencing frequent periods of dissociation whereas hyper-responsivity occurs in individuals who do not experience such periods. Their theory suggests that rather than sensory input leading to the shutdown or dissociative presentation seen, the response to sensory input is secondary to these dissociative periods. However, similar to the pattern proposed by Engel-Yeger et al. (2013), they also draw a strong connection between the two factors. An alternative rationale again for the apparently polarized sensory responses seen in trauma is that the level of responsivity relates to the type or nature of trauma experienced. Karaca Dinç et al. (2021) suggest that a pattern of hyper-responsivity to sensory input is connected with the experience of abuse and leads to hyper-vigilance, whereas hypo-responsivity is seen as resulting from neglect leading to poverty of experience, reduced opportunities to engage with their environment, and reduced sensory opportunities during important developmental periods.

Several areas of the brains of adults with childhood traumatic experiences have been found to show changes, including the hippocampus, amygdala, hypothalamus, thalamus, sensory cortex and prefrontal cortex (Cozolino, 2017; Joseph et al., 2021; Rinne-Albers et al., 2017). All of these are areas of the brain vitally important in the processing and integration of sensory input as well as the resultant skills within both emotion regulation and functioning (Harrichan et al., 2021; Holland & May-Benson, 2014). These areas are outlined in Figure 5.1. Harrichan et al. (2021) suggest that the prefrontal cortex plays a particularly important role, and that following trauma its ability to effectively integrate different senses is impaired, leaving individuals unable to form an accurate understanding of both their internal sensory experience and the world around them.

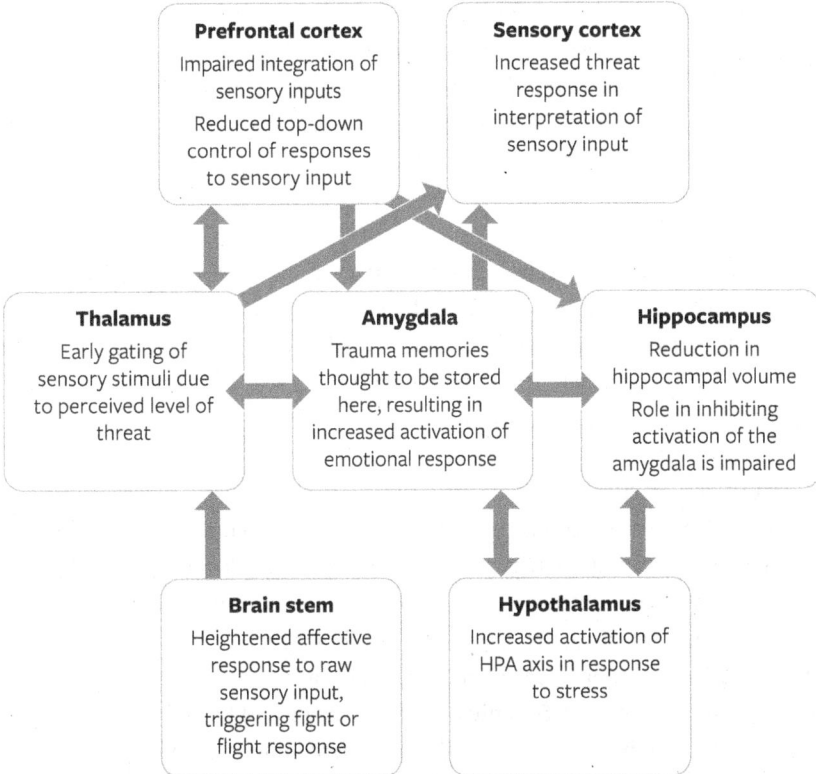

Figure 5.1 Impact of trauma on areas of the brain with a role in sensory processing and related skills (Cozolino, 2017; Engel-Yeger et al., 2013; Harricharan et al., 2021; Koomar, 2009; May-Benson, 2017)

The picture of fluctuating responsivity to sensory input identified in a number of these studies has been connected with a persistent dysregulation of the hypothalamic–pituitary–adrenal (HPA) axis, and the connected imbalance of the autonomic nervous system (ANS). This leads to individuals who have experienced trauma spending prolonged periods in fight, flight or freeze states who often present in either a state of significant hyper-arousal or overwhelm and 'shutdown' (Lehrner et al., 2016; Warner et al., 2013). A threat response or hyper-responsivity to sensory input may therefore be more apparent, with a resultant shutdown as a form of self-protection. These periods of shutdown occur when the body becomes unable to tolerate the level of perceived threat, activating the parasympathetic nervous system to the extent that a freeze response occurs (Joseph et al., 2022).

Differences in specific sensory systems

There has been some consideration in the literature of the impact of trauma on specific sensory systems, but overall, this has been small-scale in nature. Alterations that have been identified are most notable in relation to tactile, vestibular, auditory and visual processing (Engel-Yeger et al., 2013; Joseph et al., 2021; Yochman & Pat-Horenczyk, 2020).

TACTILE INPUT

The most prevalent differences reported overall have been within the tactile system, with increased impact when the trauma occurred early in childhood. This holds particular significance in view of the importance of the tactile system in the formation of attachments and regulation (Howard et al., 2020; Joseph et al., 2022; Kearney & Lanius, 2022).

VESTIBULAR SYSTEM

Changes within the vestibular system have also been frequently noted, in relation to both hyper-responsivity and hypo-responsivity (Engel-Yeger et al., 2013; McGreevy & Bolland, 2020). This is likely to have implications for sensory processing as a whole due to the role of vestibular input in the regulation and interpretation of other forms of sensory input, as well as in the development of body scheme (Kearney & Lanius, 2022). Kearney and Lanius (2022) suggest that the impaired body scheme results from detachment from the body and is a primary factor in the triggering of dissociative experiences.

SENSORY IMPACT AND THE NATURE OF THE TRAUMA

Similar to theories in relation to differing patterns of responsivity discussed above, Howard et al. (2020) discuss variations in the senses impacted according to the specific nature of the trauma. In a study using the Short Sensory Profile (Mcintosh et al., 1999), they found that children who had experienced abuse showed greater differences in relation to tactile, visual, taste/smell and auditory sensitivity, whereas children who had experienced neglect showed differences in relation to filtering of auditory information and an overall under-responsivity to sensory input. Teicher and Samson (2016) suggest further differences in relation to the type of abuse experienced, with sexual abuse being particularly connected with changes in visual and somatosensory processing.

Praxis and motor skills

The connection between trauma, sensory processing and motor skills is less well documented and perhaps less well understood, but is an important area to consider with this client group. Possible reasons for the limited available evidence could be the lack of sensory assessments for adults that are validated to assess the full spectrum of difficulties and the focus within studies having remained on modulation, with dysregulation being perceived as the primary concern. While the high level of dysregulation is significant it is likely the impact of this does not stop at sensory modulation.

Holland and May-Benson (2014) discuss the centrality of the areas of the brain that are impacted by trauma in the process of sensory integration as a whole and that this has implications beyond solely sensory modulation. They hypothesize that childhood trauma disrupts the process of sensorimotor development and praxis itself, thereby impacting an individual's coordination and body scheme (May-Benson, 2017). Teicher et al. (2016) connect these difficulties with alterations in the prefrontal cortex, an area of the brain centrally important in using sensory input to inform motor planning. As highlighted above, there is evidence to suggest that the three primary sensory systems, vestibular, proprioception and tactile, that inform the development of a motor plan, are impacted by trauma and therefore unlikely to provide sufficient information to effectively inform this ability (Matson et al., 2024). Individuals who have experienced childhood trauma have often not had the positive experiences of touch that are important in development. As a result, their ability to discriminate tactile input has not sufficiently developed and is likely to impair their fine motor skills in particular (Cox et al., 2024).

Impact of sensory processing on functioning

The pervasive nature of the physiological and emotional impact of trauma compromises both occupational performance and participation throughout the life span (Champagne & Pfeiffer, 2020; McGreevy & Bolland, 2020). The life of an individual who has experienced trauma becomes dominated by a constant need to manage their bodily responses, impacting their ability to function effectively within their environment and to engage with others. This constant automatic and involuntary response to bodily reminders of their trauma (Holland et al., 2018; Ogden et al., 2006; Van der Kolk, 2015) leads to a strong sense of disconnection or dissociation from their bodies and constant feelings of threat in response to their internal and external environments (Harrichan et al., 2021; Ogden et al., 2006; Van der Kolk, 2015). This is why Van der Kolk (2015) suggests that the starting point in recovery is in responding to and altering this responsivity to sensory input: specifically bodily sensations.

One impact of this is an active withdrawal from social relationships and intimacy, which is suggested to be an attempt to avoid sensory stimuli that are difficult to tolerate or perceived as threatening (Engel-Yeger et al., 2015). Kearney and Lanius (2022) connect this insecure attachment pattern with the somatosensory system in particular and a lack of positive touch experiences within childhood. The implications of this difficulty in forming positive relationships are likely to be wide-ranging and significant in relation to occupational engagement, leading to a number of barriers and challenges. Another prevalent impact is on the ability to sustain concentration and emotion regulation, which has the potential for a wide-ranging impact on the ability to meaningfully engage in a range of valued occupations and roles (Champagne, 2011; Joseph et al., 2022; Kennedy, 2020).

Overall, the impact of PTSD on functioning is thought to be wide-ranging and of variable extent. This variability of difficulty experienced in completion of activities of daily living has been found to correlate to the severity of their symptomology, but not specifically to sensory processing (Punski-Hoogervorst et al., 2023). Additional factors within the difficulties experienced in relation to functioning include cognitive impairments such as memory, attention and processing speed (Punski-Hoogervorst et al., 2023).

A sensory lens on hyper-vigilance and flashbacks

It is widely acknowledged that hyper-vigilance has a sensory basis, with an individual experiencing a strong automatic reaction to sensory cues that are perceived as a threat (Harricharan et al., 2021; Kearney & Lanius, 2022; Van der

Kolk, 2015). A greater understanding of the activating mechanisms within this can be helpful to inform those working with an individual who has experienced trauma and in facilitating a supportive response. Responses to sensory cues are often activated before the individual is even aware on a conscious level that this is happening, and the apparent extremity of the response can appear incongruent to the observer who does not experience the same threat response.

Trauma is thought to be processed primarily at a somatosensory level, and so in addition to the triggering of a response in relation to external sensory input, the initial reaction the person experiences is a bodily response rather than psychological (Ogden & Fisher, 2015). Hyper-vigilance can therefore be described as being under attack from both external and internal sensory stimuli, often resulting in activation of that autonomic nervous system survival response of 'fight, flight or freeze' (Kearney & Lanius, 2022; Lehrner et al., 2016).

Flashbacks are also sensory in basis and this extends beyond solely the visual aspects, with individuals also experiencing auditory, olfactory and tactile elements of these experiences (Van der Kolk, 2015). In the same way flashbacks can be activated by sensory triggers from their environment. This is likely to lead to an individual struggling to trust the sensory cues from their environment as well as a heightened response to these inputs. It is perhaps unsurprising, therefore, that individuals who have experienced trauma often present with this fluctuating response of hyper-responsivity and shutdown.

Considerations for assessment and intervention

With the significant impact the level of emotional dysregulation and sensory dysfunction resulting from trauma has on an individual's functioning and participation, there is a clear role for occupational therapists to respond to this remit. However, while sensory-based approaches have their origin within occupational therapy, the evidence base for their application in response to trauma is in its infancy (Fraser et al., 2017; McGreevy & Bolland, 2020, 2022).

An increasing number of renowned experts around trauma are advocating that these alterations in sensory processing support the need for a 'bottom-up' approach in the treatment of trauma and explain why individuals often experience difficulties utilizing approaches with a more cognitive focus (Harrichan et al., 2021; Perry, 2006; Porges, 2009; Van der Kolk, 2015). There are a growing number of studies that consider sensory-based interventions in the treatment of trauma, with a particular focus on sensory modulation (Joseph et al., 2021; McGreevy & Bolland, 2020, 2022). This is perhaps due to the acknowledgement of sensory modulation approaches as a 'bottom-up' approach to self-regulation through utilizing sensory inputs to facilitate adaptive self-management strategies (Hollands et al., 2015).

Van der Kolk (2005) and Perry and Szalavitz (2017) advocate for the centrality of enhancing feelings of safety in the recovery process. Van der Kolk (2015) asserts that this sense of safety comes from an altered relationship with sensory experiences in their bodies, stating that 'trauma victims cannot recover until they become familiar with and befriend the sensations in their bodies' (p. 100). This is also an important starting point from the perspective of sensory processing as while an individual is perceiving sensory input as threatening, they will struggle to engage with opportunities or interventions designed to challenge and develop more effective sensory perception or discrimination (Bundy & Szklut, 2020).

In order to effectively inform intervention a comprehensive assessment must be undertaken. The Adolescent/Adult Sensory Profile (Brown & Dunn, 2002) has been used in studies with this client group and is an effective tool to capture variations in sensory modulation, making this a potentially helpful starting point for the assessment process (Engel-Yeger et al., 2013; Serafini et al., 2016). However, this will not capture changes outside of this specific area and therefore it may be best to consider a tool that evaluates a wider spectrum of changes such as the Adult/Adolescent Sensory History (May-Benson, 2015).

The completion of an assessment can actually be seen as the start of the intervention process as this can begin to normalize the experiences of an individual with a trauma history. Individuals who experience trauma often display a sense of self-blaming and judgement that includes a sense of shame over their automatic responses to sensory input (Ogden et al., 2006), and completion of an assessment can help provide a rationale for what they may have been experiencing for years but without an explanation. Increased awareness and understanding of these responses can also start to increase the sense of control an individual feels in relation to those reactions and therefore help them begin to increase their ability to regulate these responses.

An important consideration in the intervention process is the experience of hyper-vigilance and the potential for this to be triggered inadvertently. Therefore, when completing sensory work with an individual who has experienced trauma, you should begin by identifying at least one regulating strategy they already have so that this can be used to support grounding as needed. As discussed in Chapter 3, Borderline Personality Disorder, deep pressure touch can be potentially problematic (Koomar, 2009), and while it should not be avoided, as it can have highly effective therapeutic benefits for this client group, it is likely to be best to start with proprioceptive inputs initially.

While it is important to assess and provide intervention for difficulties in relation to sensory discrimination and praxis, the level of dysregulation often experienced in relation to sensory input requires that the intervention process commences with a focus on improved modulation and restoring feelings of safety before moving on to challenge other difficulties (Cermak & May-Benson, 2020). This is especially important with this client group due to the added psychological aspect of the modulation difficulties, which increases the complexity of what may be happening for an individual when experiencing sensory inputs that are difficult to tolerate.

Another reason to consider sensory approaches, including higher levels of intervention, specifically Ayres Sensory Integration, is that the fidelity principles of ASI as detailed in the Ayres Sensory Integration Fidelity Measure (ASIFM) (Parham et al., 2011) show a high level of parity to trauma treatment principles overall. There is a shared emphasis within several areas but in particular on establishing a sense of safety, development of therapeutic relationships, building adaptive responses, and integration of the body and mind in treatment (Parham et al., 2011; Perry and Szalavitz, 2017; Porges, 2015; Van der Kolk, 2015), suggesting potential for ASI in meeting these needs.

Strategies and approaches

An individual who has experienced trauma may potentially benefit from the full range of sensory-based interventions, from sensory strategies to more formal Ayres Sensory Integration sessions, depending on the nature and complexity of sensory processing difficulties, and as with any client group the approach taken should be informed by your assessment findings. However, this section will focus on ideas designed to support the main areas of need or priority in intervention with trauma, which include establishing a sense of safety and strategies to help manage or reduce dissociation. For consideration of how to integrate these strategies into an overall sensory plan see Chapter 10, Sensory Strategies.

Proprioceptive strategies to support feelings of safety

Van der Kolk (2015) identifies the highest priority for individuals who have experienced trauma as 'to find a sense of safety in their own bodies' (p. 96), therefore this is a highly significant focus in intervention. Establishing this sense of safety involves a mixture of providing regulating sensory inputs to help decrease hyper-responsivity as well as re-establishing a sense of connection with the body. Proprioceptive strategies, as in the list below, are generally the most effective in doing this and also tend to be the least likely strategies to be triggering for someone, and are therefore a good place to start.

- Yoga poses involving high levels of muscle stretch. The use of yoga blocks can help to increase this stretch further, which is often more regulating.
- Weight training to provide active proprioception. This also provides an opportunity to vary the level of intensity of proprioceptive input.
- Holding a plank or completing push-ups provides a way to gain proprioceptive input without the need for equipment.
- Resistance bands provide a great activity for proprioceptive input where the intensity can be easily altered by using higher-resistance bands or lengthening or shortening the band.
- Progressive muscle relaxation encourages the tensing of muscles that provides proprioception.
  - Caution may be needed in relation to versions that direct individuals to close their eyes, which can lessen feelings of safety for an individual who has experienced trauma. In addition, mention of certain body parts could be triggering.

Deep pressure touch strategies

Deep pressure touch helps to regulate sensitivity to touch but also supports overall sensory regulation. Caution may be needed due to the potential for deep pressure to be triggering for an individual who has experienced trauma (Koomar, 2009). Therefore, the focus below is on strategies where the amount of pressure received is within the individual's control and can be altered to help reduce this risk.

- Using a body/dance sock can provide tactile input that is regulating but where the individual can alter the intensity and achieve a swaddling effect. A similar effect can be obtained by swaddling using a Lycra sheet.
- Engaging in art activities using clay can provide a way to receive deep pressure touch that is responsive to the amount of pressure the individual applies and therefore more in their control.
- Hand massage or the use of handheld massage tools allows the individual to control the amount of deep pressure input they receive and makes it more predictable.
- Wearing tight clothing or layering clothing can provide a similar effect to that received from compression garments but without the added cost.
- Using a weighted blanket or shawl provides deep pressure input to varying levels depending on the weight. It is particularly important that the individual puts this on themselves so that the input remains within their control and is expected.

Vestibular strategies

With each of these strategies, it is important that the movement is linear and rhythmic for it to have a regulating effect. Caution may be needed, as when an individual is beginning to dissociate, rhythmic vestibular input such as rocking movements can encourage further dissociation and therefore should be avoided at such times.

- Using a rocking chair can provide steady vestibular input but can feel less controlled than some other forms as it can be difficult for someone to regulate the exact amount of movement.
- Bouncing on a gym ball can provide a more predictable and controlled amount of vestibular input, which often makes it easier to tolerate.
- Jumping or bouncing on a trampoline provides more intense vestibular input, which may be more alerting. However, due to the movement, this provides proprioceptive input at the same time, which can support regulation of the input.
- Yoga poses where the head is inverted such as downward dog help provide controlled levels of vestibular input.

Strategies using other sensory inputs

- Using a night light or star projector can help to provide a low level of lighting for those who struggle to sleep in the dark and can reduce levels of hyper-vigilance.
- Listening to white noise through an app or machine.
  - Individuals who have experienced trauma are often hyper-vigilant to sounds but can also find complete silence problematic. White noise helps to direct the brain away from other background noises and as a result can be soothing.

Strategies for dissociation

For individuals who experience dissociation, it is important to identify ways to achieve grounding. The provision of intense sensory inputs can be an effective way to achieve this, but be aware that these strategies should be trialled before using during a period of dissociation.

- Sniffing aromatherapy oils or scented putty: as smells are closely connected to our emotions, this makes them highly powerful in grounding but also potentially triggering, therefore caution may be needed.

- Using a spiky massage ball to provide strong tactile input can help an individual feel present in the moment and redirect attention from other sensations.
- Placing an ice cube or textured pebble in the hand can provide grounding sensory input.
- Biting into a lemon or sucking a sour sweet provides intense gustatory input to help redirect attention.
- Listening to music that the person finds regulating can support improved overall regulation.
- Eating spicy or crunchy foods can draw focus to these sensations.
- Doing wall or chair push-ups provides strong muscle input that can help an individual to feel more present in their body.

CASE STUDY – Sofia
Background

Sofia, a 34-year-old with a diagnosis of complex PTSD, was an inpatient in a mental health treatment unit. Before going into hospital Sofia had been living on her own in a flat, which allowed her to control the level of sensory input within her environment, and she found the change to a shared environment that is much less predictable highly unsettling. Sofia had been completing a part-time job that involved mainly working from home, which suited her as there were fewer distractions. Sofia experienced high levels of hyper-vigilance and reported auditory, visual and tactile input being the most problematic for her. Sofia would spend time with a few close friends but would only agree to meet them in certain places which she was confident she would be able to tolerate.

Assessment and formulation of difficulties

In hospital Sofia struggled with a range of factors on the unit, including the bright lighting, background noises from other people, the constant opening and closing of doors, and the smells from the dining room and cleaning products. In order to sleep Sofia would leave her door open a bit to let in light from the corridor as she found it difficult to sleep in complete darkness as this increased her hyper-vigilance, but as a result she would wake up frequently in response to noises from the unit. Completion of the Adolescent/Adult Sensory Profile (Brown & Dunn, 2002) showed that Sofia experienced heightened levels of responsivity to sensory input, particularly in relation to visual, auditory, olfactory and tactile input.

Intervention

Sofia worked with her occupational therapist to help identify strategies to support her regulation and ability to manage potential triggers. Strategies initially focused on improving her sleep and altering the environment of her bedroom to support this. Sofia was provided with a small star projector that provided some light and allowed her to close her door when trying to sleep. To help reduce her reactivity to noises from the unit Sofia began using a white noise app which drew her attention away from other background noises.

Sofia also added in regulating strategies as part of her morning personal hygiene routine to help her feel more regulated at the beginning of the day. This included using a body puff to provide deeper tactile input when showering and using an electric toothbrush to provide calming vibration. She also added in products that contained scents she found regulating such as coconut-scented shower gel. Sofia also began completing a short yoga exercise before going out onto the ward to help reduce her levels of arousal. Alongside this she created a sensory kit containing items to help her feel more grounded when she felt herself becoming triggered, including sour sweets, scented putty that released an aroma as she squeezed it, and a spiky massage ball she could roll up and down her arm to feel more present.

CONCLUSION/KEY LEARNING

This chapter considers the evidence in relation to sensory processing changes in connection with trauma and how this might connect with experiences such as hyper-vigilance, flashbacks and dissociation.

Key points

- Trauma has been suggested to interrupt the process of sensory integration, with varying impacts connected to the timing and nature of the trauma experienced.
- These sensory impacts can lead to challenges in social engagement, functioning and emotion regulation.
- Sensory-based interventions can support increased feelings of safety and grounding.

CHAPTER 6

Affective and Anxiety Disorders

LEANNE DUGGAN AND REBECCA MATSON

Affective disorders are a group of mental health conditions otherwise known as mood disorders. The most frequently considered affective disorders include depression and bipolar disorder, where an individual experiences periods of both mania and depression, potentially alongside psychotic symptoms (APA, 2013). These conditions have a significant regulatory component, which suggests there is an important need to consider factors that impact on state of arousal, such as sensory processing. This chapter provides an overview of how sensory processing may be altered within these conditions but also how understanding this impact may better inform assessment and intervention and help to achieve improved outcomes.

Anxiety will be considered alongside these disorders due both to the frequent occurrence of this as a symptom of, and comorbidity with, these conditions and the significant impact this comorbidity can have on experience of these conditions and their impact on overall functioning (National Institute for Health and Care Excellence (NICE), 2014, 2022). Sensory processing challenges have been suggested to have a substantial impact on anxiety levels in relation to increasing the level of dysregulation experienced but also potentially to be the instigating factor in this element of these conditions. In order to successfully engage with our environments and function well we need to be regulated, and managing our response to sensory input is central to achieving this. This chapter will consider how understanding the implications of sensory processing can better support working with this client group and improved functional outcomes.

Alterations in sensory processing
Neurological threshold

A number of studies have considered the sensory processing patterns of individuals with depression and bipolar disorder, with the majority evaluating these two conditions together to identify the variations in symptomology and presentation apparent between the two. Overall, hypo-responsivity to sensory input, specifically the pattern identified by Dunn (2007) as low registration, where individuals have a high threshold for sensory input and a passive response, has been found to correspond with higher rates of depressed mood in both depression and bipolar disorder (Engel-Yeger et al., 2018; Khodabakhsh & Cheong, 2017; Serafini et al., 2017). Serafini et al. (2017) suggest this is evident in lower levels of motivation and an often decreased level of engagement with their environment amongst those experiencing depression. In connection with this, levels of sensation seeking, where an individual has a high threshold for sensory input and actively seeks it (Dunn, 2007), have been found to be reduced in comparison to the general population, again potentially reinforcing this withdrawn presentation (Engel-Yeger et al., 2018). It is not surprising, therefore, that higher levels of sensory seeking have been suggested to be a potential protective factor against high levels of depressive symptoms and support development of resilience, as an individual who is frequently seeking additional sensory input is much more likely to demonstrate active engagement with their environment and with other people (Serafini et al., 2017).

Dean et al. (2018) framed sensory seeking in adults as an 'active coping mechanism', where an individual is seeking out opportunities for sensations that support their self-regulation. From this perspective, using sensory-based and sensory-informed strategies as a component of a relapse prevention plan may be useful to support improved regulation and mental wellbeing. Additionally, this approach helps to empower clients to participate in their own recovery by engaging in activities and tasks that promote function through sensory regulation.

High levels of hyper-responsivity, sensory sensitivity and sensation avoiding have also been found to be much higher in affective disorders as a whole than in the general population (Engel-Yeger & Dunn, 2011; Khodabakhsh & Cheong, 2017; Serafini et al., 2017). Both sensory sensitivity and sensation avoiding relate to low thresholds for sensory input, but with sensitivity relating to a passive response and avoiding relating to an active response to managing this (Dunn, 2007). Hyper-responsivity has been connected with higher rates of anxiety, both in affective and anxiety disorders, and is suggested to lead to individuals becoming overwhelmed in different environments and social situations, resulting in withdrawal and avoidance (Hofmann & Bitran, 2007; Khodabakhsh & Cheong, 2017). Paquet et al. (2022) found that individuals with depression who displayed high levels of sensory sensitivity were 1.2 times more likely to experience anxiety, suggesting this pattern can have significant implications for experience of the condition and provide increased challenges in relation to emotion regulation.

There is a lack of clarity over whether specific sensory processing patterns lead to an individual being more susceptible to developing affective or anxiety disorders, but what is apparent is that levels of responsivity can impact on lived experience of the conditions and potentially on the overall trajectory of the condition. While there is very limited research on the influence of affective disorders on sensory discrimination and praxis, it is clear that meaningful participation in occupations and tasks changes as a component of illness (Spangler, 2011). Reduction in sensory opportunities is a complication resulting from this alteration in engagement, as is reduced access to regulating environments. This may further compound mental health symptoms by removing strategies and sensory inputs that the client relies on (whether consciously or not) to assist with achieving and maintaining regulation as a support to engagement.

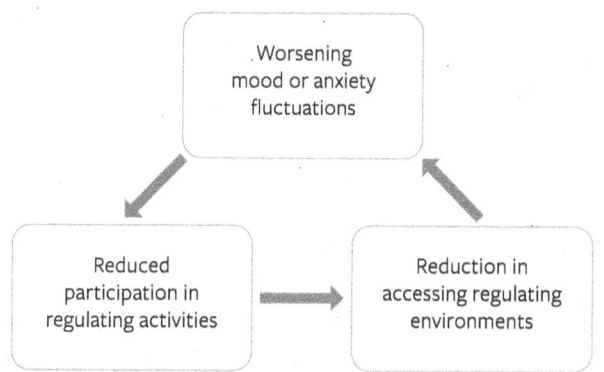

Figure 6.1 Affective disorders and their impact on access to regulation

This cycle of symptoms influencing activity choice and access to opportunities for sensory regulation, as illustrated in Figure 6.1, is a core consideration when working with this client group as it presents an opportunity from a sensory perspective to work with the client to promote regulation and function, particularly when their symptoms cause distress.

Whether sensory processing difficulties are a factor that increases an individual's vulnerability to developing depression or anxiety, occur as a result of living with either of these, or are a comorbid occurrence, supporting an individual to develop an understanding of their sensory patterns and response and ways to manage these is likely to be of benefit in both supporting emotion regulation and maintaining engagement in valued occupations.

Differences in specific sensory systems

Most studies considering sensory processing in relation to affective and anxiety disorders have focused on overall patterns of responsivity rather than reactions within the specific sensory systems, but there is some evidence for certain sensations being affected to a greater level than others. Parker et al. (2017) identified self-reported differences for individuals with bipolar disorder in relation to olfactory, gustatory, visual, tactile and auditory processing, with these changes being particularly evident or heightened during a manic phase of their condition.

TACTILE INPUT

One of the greatest areas of difference reported was tactile processing, with many experiencing increased sensitivity within this system during a manic phase, but a more varied picture of responsivity during periods of depression with some reporting experiencing decreased sensitivity. This increased sensitivity to tactile input has also been found to be present with unipolar depression, but with anxious depression in particular (Peng et al., 2019). Peng et al. (2019) link this to alterations in the areas of the brain connected with emotion regulation, and more specifically with increased grey matter volume in the post-central gyrus. They suggest this may manifest in increased hyper-vigilance in response to somatosensory input.

Paquet et al. (2022) analysed the patterns for individuals with major depressive disorder using the Adolescent/Adult Sensory Profile (Brown & Dunn, 2002), identifying that the level of responsivity seen varied between different sensations. In comparison to the norm, they found higher levels of low registration in relation to olfactory, gustatory and auditory processing; higher levels of sensory sensitivity in relation to tactile, movement, visual and auditory processing; and higher levels of sensation avoidance in response to visual, tactile and auditory input. Reduced levels of sensation seeking were particularly apparent in relation to movement, which correlated with high levels of psychomotor retardation, that is, a slowing in thought and physical movements. Paquet et al. (2022) hypothesize that the low levels of movement seeking may be a subconscious attempt to reduce the amount of sensory stimuli experienced through decreased interaction with the environment.

AUDITORY INPUT

There has been some suggestion that an impairment in relation to sensory gating, specifically of auditory input, is experienced by individuals with bipolar disorder and that they are therefore less able to filter out irrelevant or unimportant information, leading to a higher level of distraction (Cheng et al., 2016). While some studies in their meta-analysis suggested this trait was connected with the presence or absence of psychotic symptoms, Cheng et al. (2016) concluded that this feature was present regardless of psychotic symptomology, but potentially worsened in the presence of psychotic symptoms.

VISUAL PROCESSING

Some consideration has also been given to alterations in relation to visual processing for individuals with bipolar disorder, with Shaffer et al. (2018) suggesting variations in connection with different mood states. Using functional MRI they found suggestion of decreased responsivity in the areas of the brain activated in relation to visual processing, particularly the bilateral thalami. This was evident in both manic and depressed phases, but during euthymic periods of mood there were not observable differences noted between individuals with bipolar and the control group, suggesting that the fluctuations in mood experienced in this condition impact upon sensory perception within this system.

The window of tolerance and the hypothalamic–pituitary–adrenal (HPA) axis

Both affective and anxiety disorders are characterized by alterations in arousal levels that impact on ability to engage in meaningful occupations and alter sensory perception and responsivity. The window of tolerance, conceived by Siegel (1999) to conceptualize the relationship between arousal state, level of functioning and mental state, may be a helpful starting point in understanding this further. Three states of arousal are typically considered when explaining the window of tolerance. These are illustrated in Figure 6.2.

Siegel (1999) suggests that fluctuations in arousal are typical for all individuals throughout the day, and that rather than residing solely in the 'optimal' state of arousal, a typical day will cause most people to tip into both hyper- and hypo-arousal states based on exposure to stressors in the environment. Individuals with affective or anxiety disorders often spend prolonged periods in either hyper- or hypo-arousal, making it difficult to engage in their daily occupations.

There are two well-known pathways that have been connected to these fluctuations, which activate in the presence of an environmental stressor: the

HPA axis and the sympathetic nervous system (SNS) (Barel et al., 2018). These pathways developed over time as part of our safety circuity, and their primary function is to ensure our survival. The HPA axis is a series of complex endocrine mechanisms that culminate in the release of cortisol. Short-term exposure to cortisol tends to be helpful, enhancing memory and increasing energy (Cozolino, 2017). However, chronic activation of the HPA axis, such as occurs in both anxiety and depression, leads to an exaggerated stress response that becomes detrimental when not needed to escape a threat (Bear et al., 2020). Alongside this process, activation of the SNS results in physiological preparation to ensure survival, increasing availability of oxygen and glucose to fight or flee, while decreasing enervation to mechanisms that would not be a priority to ensure survival (e.g. digestion). These pathways are both reliant on the availability and activation of norepinephrine, which results in heightened arousal levels (Gunnar & Quevedo, 2007 in Lane, 2020b).

Hyper-arousal
Increasing level of alertness, which impacts negatively on:
Task performance
Social engagement
Access to language skills
Executive functioning

Optimal arousal
Often described as a 'calm/alert' state of being:
Tasks are completed
Concentration, attention and focus are optimal to support engagement with tasks

Hypo-arousal
Decreased level of alertness, which impacts negatively on:
Motivation
Task engagement
Executive functioning skills

Figure 6.2 Window of tolerance (based on Siegel, 1999)

Acknowledging these physiological processes as part of our clinical reasoning is essential when considering sensory processing in relation to affective disorders. While the core function of increased arousal is to ensure our safety in the presence of a perceived threat, it can be detrimental if activated when not needed. Sensory over-responsivity in affective disorders has been suggested to be related to this heightened functioning of the stress response system (Lane, 2020b). Repeated activation of this stress response results in a more pronounced reaction, leading to decreased feelings of safety even when not experiencing an immediate threat. The resultant increased focus on detection of threats leads to higher-order cortical functions (e.g. language, executive functioning) being 'overridden' in order to focus on ensuring safety.

Considering the impact of our arousal state in relation to the window of tolerance helps identify how alterations in the level of arousal in response to perceived environmental threats or stressors might map onto the challenges demonstrated by individuals with anxiety or affective disorders. Using the window of tolerance as a therapeutic tool with clients can assist them to conceptualize their internal experiences and empower them to understand the relationship between their arousal patterns, potential stressors and mental health symptoms.

This also helps us understand the relationship between altered sensory responsiveness and the underlying neurological processes. Without adequate regulation of arousal, the client will be inhibited by their own nervous system from engaging therapeutically with interventions or approaches that rely on the use of executive functioning skills. Using cognitive-driven resources and interventions may not be useful, and may reinforce a perceived lack of safety, as their attempts to progress with treatment are not successful. By acknowledging the innate relationship between feeling safe, modulation of arousal levels and sensory processing we can use our knowledge of how to promote function using the underlying neuroscience as a core component of our skillset.

Impact on functioning

From much of the literature, it is unclear whether the presence of sensory processing differences in affective and anxiety disorders precedes or follows the onset of the condition, but what is apparent is that the presence of altered sensory processing can have a significant impact on the experience of these conditions, their overall impact and potentially their progression as well as upon overall quality of life (Serafini et al., 2016). While not directly related to functioning, there is a suggestion that both sensory hypo-responsivity and sensory hyper-responsivity have been linked with altered experiences of symptomology that may then lead to impairments in functioning.

Sensory processing patterns have been connected with a number of traits that can impact on an individual's level of functioning and independence. Patterns of low registration have been connected with reduced motivation, and sensory sensitivity with increased anxiety, both of which may lead to a withdrawal from social engagement and impact on maintenance of occupational engagement (Engel-Yeger & Dunn, 2011). Sensory sensitivity has been connected with higher levels of negative thinking and self-blame, with a suggestion that this may be due to heightened reactions to perceived stimuli within an individual's environment (Khodabakhsh & Cheong, 2017). If we link this to how the sympathetic nervous system (SNS) and the HPA axis are activated, we can identify how sensory sensitivity, increased level of arousal and the impact of the perceived threats influence and incite perceived behaviours at a neurological level.

Wright (2020) described how this pattern of sensitivity can result in utilization of coping strategies focused on managing the level of stimulation within the environment in order to ensure circumstances that will provide less challenge and reduce unpredictability. This is likely to have a significant impact on an individual's pattern of occupational engagement overall. Additionally, depending on the nature of the experience, it may result in the individual limiting access to potentially regulating sources of sensory stimulation as they provide a level of challenge that falls outside of their window of tolerance. Through supporting individuals to increase their window of tolerance, occupational engagement is actively promoted as strategy to support access to regulatory sources of sensory input, thereby contributing to a reduction in the stress response.

Overall one of the biggest impacts on functioning suggested for individuals with anxiety and elevated levels of sensory sensitivity has been social isolation (Kinnealey & Fuiek, 1999; Wallis et al., 2018). This withdrawal or avoidance of social situations, thought to be due to their increased unpredictability or the increased demand placed on the client, will have a substantial impact on an individual's occupational engagement overall and is likely to lead to increased participation in solitary or sedentary occupations as a result.

Consider anxiety-related conditions such as agoraphobia and how these can provide an effective strategy to manage the potential for high levels of unpredictable sensory input. Being able to control the levels of input within the environment is often the most effective way to reduce anxiety levels, and individuals will often implement strategies to manage the level of sensory input without being consciously aware these inputs are a triggering factor. Intervention should aim to assist clients to become aware of how and why this may be occurring in order to develop alternative, more adaptive, ways to achieve regulation.

Supporting an individual to better understand the impact of sensory factors on their anxiety in different situations is likely to positively impact on their ability to progress within interventions that entail graded exposure as well as providing strategies to support regulation. Use of sensory modulation approaches has been found to enable improved regulation and increased participation for individuals with anxiety in situations such as use of public transport where it had previously been unmanageable (Wallis et al., 2018).

Medication and sensory processing

It has been suggested that responsivity to certain treatments, specifically antidepressants, for both individuals with depression and those with bipolar disorder may vary according to an individual's sensory profile, and there is a need to consider and account for this within the treatment process (Engel-Yeger et al., 2018). While not directly related to functioning, medication can often allow improved periods of functioning due to symptom reduction, thereby facilitating increased opportunity for engagement with a wider range of sensory opportunities.

From a therapeutic perspective, understanding the intended consequences of medication is useful when working with clients with sensory processing challenges. Identification of alterations of patterns of sensory integration dysfunction may be attributable to the timing, dosage or nature of medications prescribed and should be considered as a potential confounding factor where indicated. In their study on the relationship between sensitivities in sensory processing and sensitivity to medication, Jagiellowicz et al. (2024) identified moderate significant correlations between sensory processing sensitivity and response to medication across three adult participant groups (range: 18–81 years). They suggest that this relationship requires further research to consider how it could inform medication dosage, potential effectiveness and adverse drug reaction. There is also the potential that medication sensitivity could be an indicator of sensory hypersensitivity in the clinical population.

Sleep and sensory processing

There is currently limited evidence on the relationship between sleep, sensory processing and impact on functional capacity. However, sleep is an area thought to be particularly susceptible to the impact of sensory sensitivity for those with generalized anxiety disorder (Khodarahimi et al., 2021). Khodarahimi et al. (2021) identified that while negative affect in itself could impact upon the experience of dreams and sleep quality, this was significantly higher in those identified as experiencing heightened sensory sensitivity. Altered sleep quality is often an area of concern within affective and anxiety disorders, therefore an understanding of how sensory processing can impact on this experience could be of importance in effectively intervening in this area of daily life and supporting the development of effective strategies for self-management. De Lecea et al. (2012) suggest that as difficulties in maintaining arousal states including sleep have been associated with various mental health difficulties, including anxiety and depression, understanding the neurobiological factors that underpin these changes could help to explain why levels of vigilance, sensory responsivity and emotion regulation are also altered.

In the general population poor quality sleep has been found to significantly correlate with sensory sensitivity and sensory avoiding, with heightened tactile and auditory responsivity being the biggest factors within this (Engel-Yeger & Shochat, 2012). Therefore when working with individuals experiencing sleep difficulties, evaluation of their sensory processing patterns is likely to be an important part of the process. If clients are able to access good quality, restful sleep, this provides a clear foundation on which to build the rest of their day. Identifying strategies that support appropriate alterations of arousal across a 24-hour period also provides a clear foundation on which to build their sensory and emotional wellbeing.

A sensory lens on anxiety

The connection between sensory processing and our arousal levels has long been acknowledged within the sensory integration literature, but the extent of this is perhaps only just being fully realized outside of occupational therapy. While it is unclear if heightened levels of sensory sensitivity precede or follow the onset of anxiety disorders, it is evident that sensory triggers can escalate levels of existing anxiety and cause an increase in arousal state. When in a state of heightened anxiety, the brain becomes hyper-focused on cues of potential danger, creating a state of hyper-vigilance. The result of this is that the brain is constantly scanning the environment for danger and is more likely to respond to changes or information that would otherwise usually be filtered out as irrelevant by the brain, which will impact on the client's capacity to access a range of cognitive skills, in addition to placing limitations on engagement in occupations that do not work towards maintaining safety. Over time, this is where we can see changes in the level of function across a range of occupational domains, as the human nervous system is hardwired to prioritize safety above all other goals.

Registering of sensory cues from the environment often occurs on a subconscious level and this can lead to a gradual increase in arousal levels over the day to the point where this suddenly becomes overwhelming without that person being aware how it reached that point. This can seem to an observer as if that person has been triggered disproportionately by one particular sensory event, when it actually may be an accumulation of factors across a period of time during the day. Even for an individual with no significant sensory processing difficulties, this element of reactivity will exist and impact upon their overall regulation.

Panic attacks, for example, are often triggered before the person is even aware of the trigger or cue for their sudden increase in anxiety, and sensory factors, both interoceptive and exteroceptive, can play a significant part in this. The symptoms experienced during a panic attack have been connected to altered sensory perception and processing, with a suggested connection to the parietal gyrus; however, further research is needed to confirm this (Zhou et al., 2022). Interoceptive signals are of great significance as indicators of activation of the SNS when experiencing panic, including palpitations, dizziness, shortness of breath, feelings of disembodiment, a sense of impending doom and pain or discomfort (Elias et al., 2020; Khalsa & Feinstein, 2019). Considering potential sensory cues that may instigate a panic attack and identifying strategies to manage this are likely to be a highly important part of intervention as a way of empowering clients to combat their potential avoidance of anxiety-provoking situations.

The limbic system, and particularly the amygdala, is central in both our experience of anxiety and in regulating our response to sensations and modulating the responsivity of the autonomic nervous system – including activation of the SNS (Bear et al., 2020). Dysregulation of the amygdala leads to difficulty in regulating our emotional responses and it is likely that avoidant responses to sensory input are a result of negative tagging of those sensations in the amygdala (Lane, 2020b). This is a concern when considering interoceptive functioning, as fear of experiencing these physical, interoceptive signals of anxiety may further increase the level of arousal, with further impact on the ability of the client to engage in their routine and meaningful occupations.

Overall there is thought to be a bidirectional relationship between dysregulation of the amygdala and avoidant responses, and identifying which is the causal factor may be difficult to ascertain. The neurobiology of this process is outlined in Figure 6.3.

Regardless of the initial factor, however, sensory modulation approaches which work on a 'bottom-up' approach are likely to support the necessary down-regulation to enable an individual to achieve and maintain an arousal state which supports their ability to engage and participate meaningfully in their valued occupations.

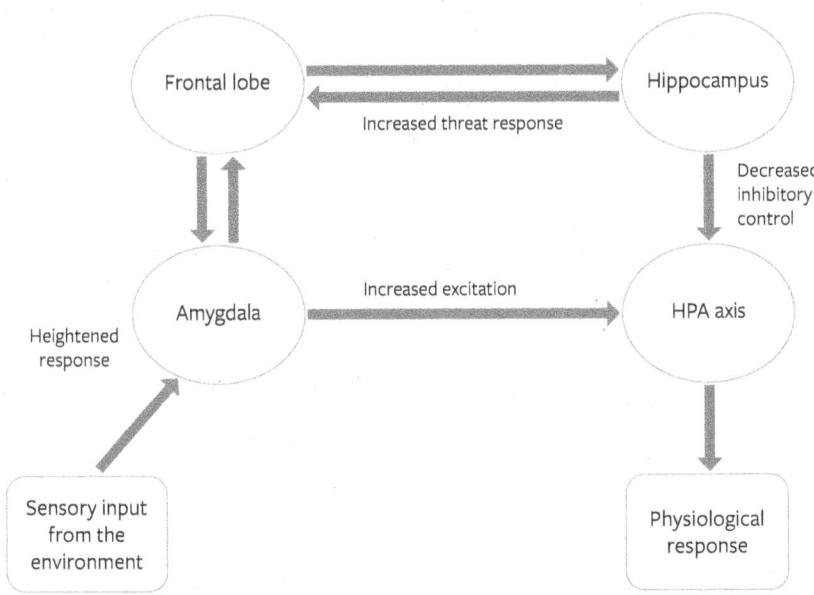

Figure 6.3 Impact of sensory input on neurobiological response to anxiety

Considerations for assessment and intervention

When working with individuals with affective disorders there may need to be an awareness that response to sensory input may or may not be a stable trait and, particularly with bipolar disorder, that the level of responsivity could alter depending on the mood state at different times. This is likely to create an added complexity to the assessment process and a potential need to identify alternative strategies or approaches depending on mood state at the time.

Sensory modulation has frequently been used as an approach to support regulation of arousal levels and therefore could be considered a particularly suitable approach for affective and anxiety disorders where there can be significant and rapid changes in arousal state. The first step towards developing such plans may be to gain a deeper understanding not only of how an individual's mood fluctuates in general but also how different sensory inputs may increase or instigate these fluctuations.

Approaches to assessment

The Adolescent/Adult Sensory Profile (Brown & Dunn, 2002) has been used in a number of studies to identify the sensory processing patterns of individuals with depression and bipolar disorder, and could be considered particularly suitable due to the focus on modulation and the regulatory response to sensory input. Individuals with bipolar disorder were also one of the client groups used as a comparison in development of the norms for this assessment (Pearson Education, 2019). While this assessment only considers modulation, this is the primary area of sensory processing difficulty that has been identified within bipolar disorder and anxiety disorders, so this may be sufficient.

However, there is some suggestion of impairments in sensory perception also in relation to auditory gating and visual perception, and therefore more comprehensive evaluation may be necessary, which could be supported by an assessment such as the Adult/Adolescent Sensory History (May-Benson, 2015) that also considers sensory discrimination and motor skills. Another potential benefit of this assessment when working with individuals with affective and anxiety disorders is that this assessment also provides scores in relation to 'social/emotional' in the context of these difficulties.

Another useful assessment to consider is the Multidimensional Assessment of Interoceptive Awareness, Version 2 (MAIA-2) (Mehling et al., 2018) as this provides clients with the opportunity to reflect on their processing of interoceptive signals and identify if they may be impacting on their increased arousal state. Further information on this assessment is available in Chapter 8, Assessment and Goal Setting.

These assessments are primarily client-rated rather than objectively rated clinician-administered assessments. Some assessment questions can be interpreted in a number of ways, which the client may or may not identify with. From a sensory formulation perspective, it may be useful to complete the assessments with the client to ensure the data collected is representative of their experience. Additionally, this allows the therapist the opportunity to build rapport, and to gather additional qualitative information to add to their clinical reasoning process.

Strategies and approaches
Sensory support plans, sensory diet and sensory-focused routines

Sensory support plans can be of value not only in providing strategies to support maintenance of overall arousal levels but also to provide 'in the moment' strategies when encountering unexpected triggers. These can be accompanied by a sensory kit containing items that support the plan to create ease of access and a physical prompt to use the strategies when needed. A plan is likely to include a mix of strategies to increase and decrease arousal states but may focus much more on one than the other depending on the current level of dysregulation. Sensory plans and kits are explained in more detail in Chapter 10, Sensory Strategies, and may be of use in conjunction with the client-group-specific considerations within this chapter. With an individual with high levels of depression there will be a much greater focus on strategies to increase arousal while with higher levels of anxiety there will be a greater need for those that decrease arousal levels. In the case of bipolar disorder, a more complex form of intervention planning may be required so as to include strategies which are reflective of their fluctuations in mood. Depending on the level of insight of the client when their mood is elevated, it may be necessary to include others such as family members or supporting staff in the creation of the intervention plan. Their function would be to promote and encourage access to sources of sensory input that may assist with regulation of arousal and subsequent capacity to engage in meaningful activity.

Considerations when identifying specific sensory strategies

Sensory strategies can be broadly defined as those that are commonly calming or alerting. However, you may find different reactions to those expected from your clients. This is where taking time to understand an individual's sensory patterns prior to suggesting strategies or interventions can help guide you and them to find the most suitable strategies.

This is also an opportunity to engage in client-led practice, whereby the client actively contributes to the structure and content of their plan by advising the therapist of their sensory preferences and experiences. This process is superimposed over the knowledge you have gained as part of your assessment process, where you have obtained a baseline picture of the client's presentation and sensory responses so as to create an individualized, impactful, sensory-informed plan of support to assist with their mental health recovery.

Strategies to decrease arousal

These strategies have been identified as being commonly experienced as calming. The purpose of these strategies is to decrease the level of arousal experienced by the client, and to increase their functional capacity and their ability to engage meaningfully with their daily routine. They have been separated into the different sensory systems for ease of identification.

> **Note:** A certain amount of trial and error will be required to identify those which are effective for each client as each person processes

sensation in a unique manner. Additionally, these strategies should be identified and implemented within the context of an overall plan to support regulation. Isolated strategy use will not be as effective as building opportunities for regulation into the client's daily routine.

VESTIBULAR AND PROPRIOCEPTIVE STRATEGIES

- Yoga or tai chi poses with high levels of muscle stretch.
- Progressive muscle relaxation.
- Lifting weights.
- Body-weight exercises like holding a plank, doing push-ups.
- Doing wall or chair push-ups.
- Gardening activities that involve digging.
- Cooking or baking activities that involve kneading, such as making bread or pizza dough.
- Slow, linear movement such as sitting on a swing and moving slowly.

TASTE AND OLFACTORY STRATEGIES

- Smelling aromatherapy oils such as lavender or vanilla.
- Regulation through food like chewing gum or chewy sweets, or eating crunchy foods like pretzels, crisps, apples.
- Drinking warm milky drinks can support a decrease in arousal both due to the warmth providing a calming sensation and milk containing tryptophan, an amino acid thought to support regulation of arousal (Singh, 2016).

TACTILE STRATEGIES
These strategies are deep-touch pressure-based strategies.

- Using weighted items such as a weighted blanket, weighted shawl or weighted animal.
- Hand massage or using massage balls.
- Using fidget tools such as a tangle fidget or stress ball.
- Wearing tight clothing such as fitted jeans or Lycra can be a good way to gain deep pressure touch.
- Deep breathing exercises.

- Using a hot water bottle is useful both in terms of providing deep pressure tactile stimulation as well as providing thermostimulation.

VISUAL STRATEGIES

- Dimmed lighting can help to reduce the level of visual stimulation, and thereby decrease arousal levels.
- Changing lightbulbs from bright white to a more yellow tone to reduce glare.
- Using a night light as an alternative to the main lighting.
- A fibre optic lamp can also provide lower levels of lighting.
- Wearing sunglasses to reduce brightness of external environments.

AUDITORY STRATEGIES

- Listening to white noise can help focus attention away from other background noises.
- Listening to music with a steady beat.
- Wearing over-ear headphones or ear defenders when overwhelmed.

Strategies to increase arousal

These strategies have been identified as being commonly experienced as alerting. The purpose of these strategies is to increase the level of arousal experienced by the client, to increase their functional capacity and their ability to engage meaningfully with their daily routine. They have been separated into the different sensory systems for ease of identification.

> **Note:** A certain amount of trial and error will be required to identify those that are effective for each client as each person processes sensation in a unique manner. Additionally, it is important to build the client's level of understanding of their sensory processing needs and identifying signs of being within their window of tolerance. Inappropriate use of strategies that increase arousal may result in too significant an increase in the level of arousal. It is therefore important to discuss indications for use, timing, frequency and duration of engagement in the below strategies to ensure optimal therapeutic results.

VESTIBULAR AND PROPRIOCEPTIVE STRATEGIES

- Dancing: fast and spinning movements tend to be the most alerting as they provide higher levels of vestibular input. The impact on arousal levels may therefore need to be monitored more closely initially.
- Using a trampette or trampolining can be a good way to provide vestibular and proprioceptive input together. Receiving proprioceptive input at the same time helps that individual regulate the sensory input and reduces the risk of it becoming overloading.
- Going for a run helps to provide both of these inputs but in a way that is more easily controlled by the individual as they can alter the pace or choose to run on the flat or an incline, thereby altering the level of these inputs they receive.

TASTE AND OLFACTORY STRATEGIES

- Sucking on sour sweets.
- Biting into a lemon.
- Drinking an icy/cold drink.
- Smelling aromatherapy oils or scented products such as peppermint, eucalyptus and citrus scents, which tend to be alerting.

TACTILE STRATEGIES

- Fidgeting with a koosh ball.
- Plunging a hand into mixed materials, rice or beans.
- Having a cold shower.
- Holding an ice cube or ice pack.
- Using a loofah or body puff as part of their personal hygiene routine.

VISUAL STRATEGIES

- Bright lighting provides increased stimulation and is more awakening.
- Wearing colourful clothing can also be helpful in a similar way.

AUDITORY STRATEGIES

- Listening to fast-paced music or music with an irregular beat.

- Listening to audio books or podcasts can also provide alerting auditory input.
- Choosing to work in a busy environment that provides low-level background noise can be alerting in a helpful way for some people.
- Having the TV on in the background can be helpful for some people.

CASE STUDY – Remi
Background
Remi, 42 years old, had an established diagnosis of anxiety disorder. Remi was referred to occupational therapy services to assist with returning to work following a period of decreased functioning due to an exacerbation of anxiety symptoms. During the initial interview Remi reported feeling overwhelmed by everything and noted difficulties identifying when anxiety was building until it was unmanageable. Remi was finding existing strategies to manage anxiety ineffective due to difficulties engaging with them. Remi indicated becoming actively distressed at times, particularly due to noises in their environment, so would avoid loud or unpredictable environments.

Assessment and formulation of difficulties
Completion of the Adolescent/Adult Sensory Profile (Brown & Dunn, 2002) found that Remi scored less than most people in relation to low registration and sensation seeking, and more than most for sensory sensitivity, particularly in relation to tactile and auditory input, and sensory avoiding across all senses. The Multidimensional Assessment of Interoceptive Awareness, Version 2 (MAIA-2) (Mehling et al., 2018) was also completed with Remi, which showed increased sensitivity to interoceptive input. This included difficulties distracting themselves from uncomfortable sensations, and worrying and emotional distress due to internal sensations, resulting in decreased reliance on body signals as a source of information or as a tool to promote regulation, and decreased feelings of safety and trust in their internal body signals. A hypothesis was identified that Remi's difficulties with social engagement and avoidance of interpersonal environments were due to hyper-responsivity in the tactile, auditory and interoceptive systems.

Intervention
Intervention focused on creating a sensory-enhanced routine that promoted Remi's ability to engage with external environments and identifying sensory

strategies that would help decrease their level of arousal. Education was also provided to promote Remi's understanding and awareness of how their sensory processing influences their mental health, and to empower them to identify strategies.

CONCLUSION/KEY LEARNING

This chapter considers the evidence relating to sensory processing patterns in connection with affective disorders, including anxiety, depression and bipolar disorder. Responsivity has been suggested to vary between these conditions, with heightened responsivity being more apparent in anxiety and reduced responsivity in connection with depression.

Key points

- The window of tolerance may be a helpful tool to understand fluctuations in arousal with this client group, and how sensory inputs could lead to these fluctuations.
- Sensory inputs can be used therapeutically to facilitate movement between arousal levels to enable engagement.

CHAPTER 7

Dementia

LEANNE DUGGAN AND REBECCA MATSON

Dementia is an umbrella term used to describe 'a syndrome, usually of a chronic or progressive nature, caused by a variety of brain illnesses that affect memory, thinking, behaviour and ability to perform everyday activities' (World Health Organization (WHO), 2021). This is a complex area of clinical practice, which encompasses a range of neurological conditions, and while it is not classified as a mental health condition, individuals who experience dementia often receive treatment from mental health professionals and within mental health services, therefore consideration has been given to dementia within this book.

Dementia entails both cognitive and behavioural impacts including memory difficulties, personality changes, alterations in communication and reduced ability to complete daily tasks (NICE, 2018). The most commonly identified forms of dementia include Alzheimer's disease (60%–70% of cases); vascular dementia (10%–20% of cases); frontotemporal dementia (10% of cases); and Lewy body dementia (5% of cases) (Dementia UK, 2024; Lad et al., 2022).

The number of people being diagnosed with dementia is increasing and is expected to continue to do so due to an ageing population, making identifying ways to support and improve the quality of life for this client group of increasing necessity. Changes to the structures of the brain as dementia progresses understandably influence the ability of the person to integrate sensation in a way that allows them to meet the demands of their tasks or environments (Behrman et al., 2014). Using a sensory approach with clients with a diagnosis of dementia provides a non-pharmacological intervention opportunity that aims to promote participation, function and comfort as their dementia progresses.

Dementia is a progressive illness which has been identified as having several stages. Depending on the source, these stages may differ slightly in their description, reflecting the wide-ranging challenges a person with dementia may experience, but aim to map out how the condition is likely to progress. One example that may be helpful is that provided by Champagne (2018) in her book *Sensory Modulation in Dementia Care*, which separates the stages into early, middle and late stages according to severity of symptoms, level of functional difficulties relating to areas such as communication, cognition and mobility, and independence in activities of daily living. Certain symptoms may progress alongside the illness, while others resolve as the dementia progresses. Symptoms have been noted to be non-linear in that some may develop in particular stages, while others may develop much later or not at all, leading to the client's presentation and needs changing as the condition progresses. This will directly influence choice of therapeutic approach, identified goals and intervention strategies.

Behavioural and psychological symptoms of dementia (BPSD) are one of the most frequent reasons for referral to mental health services. They have been described as symptoms of the 'deterioration in perception and thought content, deterioration in mood, motor activity disorders and personality changes' that are experienced as part of dementia (Özata Değerli & Altuntaş, 2023, p. 1). Symptoms are thought to be observed in up to 90 per cent of individuals with dementia (Cerejeira et al., 2012) and include psychological symptoms such as delusions, hallucinations and anxiety, and behavioural symptoms such as disinhibition, irritability and aberrant motor behaviour (Cerejeira et al., 2012; Mukherjee et al., 2017).

Aberrant motor behaviour can be defined as 'aimless movement without a specific purpose' (Dimitriou et al., 2022). From a sensory perspective, it is essential to consider the purpose of this behaviour and how it may relate to underlying sensory changes resulting in an attempt to promote regulation through movement, which may be framed in certain care settings as 'agitation' or 'restlessness'. Providing education to carers, family members and staff on the origin and purpose of this behaviour may result in increasing the client's access to movement as an opportunity for regulation.

This chapter aims to consider the specific sensory challenges relevant to individuals with dementia, and how this may indicate the relevance and potential for a sensory-based approach to intervention. Due to a high proportion of individuals with dementia falling within the older adult client group (i.e. 65 years and over), attention will also be given to sensory alterations or challenges experienced as part of the ageing process to provide further context.

Alterations in sensory processing

Healthy ageing leads to changes within the structure of the brain, resulting in alterations in function, cognition and behaviour (Spooner et al., 2021). When working within a sensory framework the primary focus is to establish the impact of sensory processing on participation (Bundy & Lane, 2020; Miller et al., 2017); therefore it is important to recognize the difference between changes due to a healthy ageing process, and those due to challenges with processing sensory information.

Older adults as a population often experience changes in relation to responsivity to sensory input primarily within the category identified by Dunn's (1997) model as low registration, suggesting a reduced response to sensory input and a high neurological threshold (Pohl et al., 2003). The levels of low registration have also been suggested to increase with age within this client group, with more significant levels of low registration being identified by Pohl et al. (2003) in those 75 years and older, leading to increased risk of sensory deprivation. Alongside this there has been some suggestion that older adults also find it more difficult to filter irrelevant sensory input. Age-related sensory changes have been suggested to put an individual at greater risk of cognitive decline and conditions such as dementia, making sensory processing of increased significance to consider, both within the general older adult population and those with dementia.

Levels of sensory seeking and sensory sensitivity have been found to reduce as part of the ageing process and this has been suggested to impact on functional skills such as hand-writing (Engel-Yeger et al., 2012). Correia et al. (2016) found that two thirds of a sample of 3005 healthy older adults experienced impairments in two or more sensory systems, with tactile discrimination identified as one of the most prevalent areas of decline. They connect this to decreased nerve conduction velocity, decreased density of tactile receptors and grey-matter changes in the central nervous system (CNS) that occur as part of the ageing process. Reduced precision of proprioceptive feedback has also been identified in older adults, impacting on praxis, specifically in relation to feedforward mechanisms that are dependent on the ability to compare predicted and actual sensory feedback from a task in order to inform motor actions (Lei & Wang, 2017). Altered sensory processing as part of the ageing process has also been connected with the increased falls risk that tends to become more apparent as the condition progresses (Zilbershlag et al., 2023).

Neurological threshold
ALTERATIONS IN DEMENTIA

As with the general population of older adults, low registration has been identified as a consistently higher factor in those with dementia (Chung, 2006; Özata Değerli & Altuntaş, 2023; Zaree et al., 2023). Zaree et al. (2023) found the level of difference with the general population to be of statistical significance (p = 0.001), and there has been some suggestion that the levels of low registration correlate with severity of dementia, but as yet this has not been fully evaluated. Özata Değerli and Altuntaş (2023) considered these differences in the context of BPSD and found higher levels of both low registration and sensory sensitivity to have a statistically significant correlation with severity of BPSD, inferring the importance of considering the impact of these alterations in order to most effectively support this client group.

Variable results have been found in relation to the other quadrants of the Adolescent/Adult Sensory Profile (AASP) (Brown & Dunn, 2002), with increased levels of sensory sensitivity identified by Özata Değerli and Altuntaş (2023) in individuals with BPSD, but lower levels of sensitivity identified by Chung (2006), and no difference found by Zaree et al. (2023). Conflicting results have also been found in relation to sensory avoiding, with two studies suggesting higher levels of avoidance (Rhodus et al., 2022; Zaree et al., 2023), one study finding no difference (Özata Değerli & Altuntaş, 2023), and one suggesting lower levels of avoidance in comparison with the general population of older adults (Chung, 2006). Levels of sensation seeking have been identified as decreasing with age by a similar amount in the general population and those with dementia (Özata Değerli & Altuntaş, 2023). These studies suggest that individuals with dementia may experience difficulties perceiving or registering sensory stimuli, as well as difficulties experiencing the stimulation they do detect as 'safe'. When sensation is experienced as unclear, unsafe or overwhelming it can alter the ability of the person to maintain an appropriate level of arousal to meet the demands of tasks and of their environment.

The differing levels of responsivity in these studies could be due to various factors, including the severity of dementia and environmental factors such as level of stimulation and physical environment (i.e. living at home, in a care home or a hospital facility). A high proportion of individuals in the above studies had the Alzheimer's form of dementia and the majority lived in the community with caregivers. Zaree et al. (2023) considered a higher number of individuals with moderate severity of dementia, which may be the reason for differences to the other studies. Another factor in variability in the results seen is differences between whether the AASP was completed by the individual themselves or by a caregiver, both of which could have implications for reliability of report. There is also substantial variation in the sample sizes within the studies, ranging from nine participants (Rhodus et al., 2022) to 130 participants (Zaree et al., 2023), so some caution may be needed when considering these results and their implications.

A number of areas integral to sensory processing are altered in connection with dementia, including the hippocampus, temporal lobe, frontal lobe and parietal lobe, with the hippocampus, which has been suggested to support sensory modulation, being one of the earliest affected areas (Fletcher et al., 2015; Lane, 2020b). How the areas of the brain first impacted varies depending on the type of dementia, and the potential implications of this on early changes in sensory processing, are considered in Table 7.1.

Table 7.1 Early areas of the brain impacted in different types of dementia and the potential impacts on sensory processing (Borghammer et al., 2021; Puppala et al., 2021; Tahami Monfared et al., 2022)

	Alzheimer's dementia	Frontotemporal dementia	Lewy body dementia
Area of the brain first affected	Hippocampus	Frontal and temporal lobes, specifically the anterior cingulate cortex	Amygdala, substantia nigra
Nature of the impact	Neuronal loss, atrophy and build-up of amyloid plaques and tau tangles	Progressive nerve cell loss and atrophy of the lobes	Neuronal loss and accumulation of Lewy bodies impacting on dopamine production
Dementia symptoms	Formation of new memories and learning Disorientation Problem-solving	Personality and behaviour Language Planning and organization Memory	Tremors and rigidity Hallucinations Concentration
Potential impact on sensory processing	Impaired filtering of sensory input Increased emotional response Difficulty matching sensory input to past experience	Inability to contextualize sensory input Impairments in auditory and visual processing Increased emotional response Altered pain perception	Impaired sensorimotor integration Difficulties integrating tactile and proprioceptive information

Vascular dementia is not included within this table as this type of dementia is caused by reduced blood flow to the brain rather than originating in one particular part of the brain. The primary areas of the brain that have been discussed within studies of altered reactivity for individuals with dementia are the temporal lobe and the limbic system (Alves et al., 2014; Fletcher et al., 2015; Zaree et al., 2023). The temporal lobe has a key role in contextualizing experience of sensory input in connection with memories and emotions, and therefore the atrophy to this area of the brain could have a significant impact on sensory reactivity and ability to effectively integrate sensory information to inform interactions and behaviour (Zaree et al., 2023). Changes in this area have been specifically linked to alternations in response to pain, temperature and olfactory input (Alves et al., 2014; Fletcher et al., 2015). This is important to consider when framing sensory processing in terms of risk, as alteration in the ability of the individual to register pain and temperature may inadvertently increase risk-taking behaviour during activities of daily living. An example of this would be reaching over a boiling pot of water to get an item overhead without due regard for the risk of burning exposed skin. In individuals with frontotemporal dementia, Fletcher et al. (2015) found changes in responsivity to also be connected with atrophy to the right mid-insula. This could link with changes to interoceptive functioning, which is discussed later in this chapter.

Differences in specific sensory systems

Changes in vision, hearing, olfaction and taste are relatively well documented within the literature for older adults, with some suggestion these areas are more significantly impacted in those with dementia (Crowe, 2014; Haigh & Mighton, 2016; Lad et al., 2022). Impairments in processing of olfactory, visual and auditory input in particular have been suggested to be a potential risk factor for later development of dementia (Dintica et al., 2019; Lad et al., 2022; Livingston et al., 2020), rather than a subsequent development due to the condition. One reason for this could be the impact of this degeneration on levels of sensory deprivation, which can lead to increased confusion and disorientation (Cusic et al., 2022; Haigh & Mighton, 2016). Jakob and Collier (2017) highlight this as a particular potential risk factor for those living in longer-term care facilities such as care homes where individuals may have minimal control over the sensory qualities of their environments, resulting in reduced levels of stimulation, or over-stimulation due to the overwhelm of increased unfamiliar sensory input.

OLFACTORY PROCESSING

Particular focus has been given to changes in olfactory processing for those with dementia and has been linked to a more rapid level of cognitive decline (Dintica et al., 2019; Lad et al., 2022). Olfactory input has the most direct pathway to the cortex, meaning this form of sensory input tends to have the quickest impact and can rapidly alter levels of arousal. Due to the direct route it has to the amygdala and hippocampus, there can be a strong emotional response to smell and it can also trigger recall of memories (Lad et al., 2022; Lane, 2020a). This is perhaps why this sensory system has received attention in the context of onset and trajectory of dementia. Estimated rates of olfactory system deterioration are thought to be as high as 100 per cent for individuals with Alzheimer's disease and 96 per cent for those with frontotemporal dementia (Alves et al., 2014). Alves et al. (2014) suggest these changes are more strongly related to discrimination, that is, making sense of the input, rather than perception of the input, but it is likely that both are impacted as part of the general ageing process (Palmquist et al., 2020).

TACTILE INPUT

Deficits have also been identified within the tactile system in relation to processing of temperature and pain in particular, but with the suggestion that this varies in prevalence according to type of dementia (Fletcher et al., 2015; Smith et al., 2023). Fletcher et al. (2015) found the most significant variations in response to pain and temperature in frontotemporal dementia: 71 per cent of people compared to 45 per cent for those with Alzheimer's disease. Altered response to temperature was more commonly reported than pain, with more of a negative reaction to cold than hot temperatures. These alterations are likely to have a significant impact on an individual's level of distress and emotion regulation, making it an important consideration for those working with this client group. Whereas in most forms of dementia an increased responsivity to pain was identified, a decreased level of responsivity was noted in frontotemporal dementia, suggesting a potential factor in some of the behavioural challenges noted (Jonsdottir & Gunnarsson, 2021).

INTEROCEPTIVE PROCESSING

Individuals with frontotemporal dementia have also been suggested to experience interoceptive overload, that is, increased awareness of internal sensations, impacting on areas such as sleep quality and enjoyment of activities (Migeot et al., 2022; Wei & Van Somermen, 2020). The insula, which is of central importance in processing interoceptive information, has shown altered signal strength in the dementia population as a whole (Birba et al., 2022). Due to the role of interoception in cognitive and emotional processing, this could result in preoccupation and high levels of distress regarding processing of interoceptive information. An example of this would be clients who present with high levels of distress or agitation due to a perceived significant need to urinate, but being physically unable to do so.

Motor skills and mobility

While it may be relevant to consider the impact of ageing on motor skills for this client group overall, this is particularly important in Lewy body dementia, where similar motor challenges to those experienced with Parkinson's disease can be seen (Lad et al., 2022). A different picture is suggested for Alzheimer's disease, where ability for motor learning is preserved overall, which is thought to be due to the differentiation in areas of the brain being impacted by progression of the different forms of dementia. Collier et al. (2010) found improvements in both motor and process skills following administration of a tailored multi-sensory environment intervention as measured using the Assessment of Motor and Process Skills (AMPS) (Fisher, 2006). They suggest this may be due to the deterioration in motor performance in dementia relating to the impact of cognitive deficits on sensory processing and motor skills rather than specific neural damage. This may be conceptualized as alterations to the routes and pathways within the brain rather than alterations to the neurological structures themselves. Therefore, providing enhanced amounts of sensory inputs has the potential to produce an improvement in this area and increase independent functioning.

The reduction often seen in overall postural stability and balance is a common co-occurrence with dementia and is thought to result from reduced communication between different areas of the brain responsible for sensory processing, specifically impairments of the parietal lobe (Ma et al., 2022; Zhang et al., 2019). There is less evidence in relation to the potential of sensory interventions such as multi-sensory environments to improve this area, with some improvement noted but not to a significant level (Cusic et al., 2022). However, in some cases the promotion of enhanced vestibular and proprioceptive opportunities through movement and the connected postural demands may provide opportunities for regulation and assist with reinforcing body boundaries. This can help to promote feelings of safety as part of an individualized sensory-informed intervention plan.

Impact of sensory processing on functioning

As mentioned above, older adults in general experience sensory loss and are at greater risk of sensory deprivation, with the risks increasing when in an environment over which they have reduced control such as a care home (Jakob & Collier, 2017). This can also lead to them being more prone to social isolation and reduced emotional wellbeing (Lad et al., 2022). Both auditory and visual impairments have been linked with heightened risk of cognitive decline and resultant decreased levels of independence in activities of daily living (Swenor et al., 2019). Alterations in olfactory detection have been suggested to have broad impacts, such as limiting food choice and preferences, reduced appetite, and safety concerns due to inability to detect food that has spoiled or dangers such as a gas leak (Alves et al., 2014; Palmquist et al., 2020). This has potential implications both for physical and emotional wellbeing.

While the decline in independent functioning often experienced by individuals with dementia is most frequently connected with the level of cognitive decline, there has been suggestion that sensory stimulation can be effectively used to improve engagement and functioning (Collier et al., 2010; Lorusso & Bosch, 2018). This may be particularly important for those residing in a care home or hospital environment due to alterations in the sensory cues that may support initiation and engagement in occupations. Bailliard (2015) describes this experience as sensory dissonance, where there is a mismatch between the sensory cues within an environment and those expected by the person, leading to increased cognitive demands within an activity, increased levels of distress and reduced motivation for engagement. Therefore for an individual with dementia who experiences increased challenges in cognitive recall, dependence on sensory cues is likely to be even greater.

This will be further compounded where alterations have occurred in their language centres, resulting in shifts in their capacity for receptive and expressive language. Potkins et al. (2003) identified links between BPSD symptoms and expressive and receptive language impairments in their study. They identified the subsequent decrease in participation in social activity and a reduction in social interactions as being of significant concern within the dementia population. Ensuring consistent access to regulating sources of sensory input may assist with decreasing frustration and symptoms of BPSD resulting from changes in language processing, as engagement is not reliant on verbal communication.

Providing appropriate levels of sensory input also supports an individual to alter their level of arousal and attention and can therefore improve levels of orientation and interaction. However, it is important to keep in mind that everyone's level of responsivity to sensory input may be different and that they may therefore require different levels of sensory input to support and regulate alertness. This is why one of the main criticisms in the evidence base for multi-sensory interventions with dementia is the lack of personalization that is often evident in spaces designed to support this.

Dementia-friendly universal design principles, such as those identified by the National Disability Authority (2015), are useful when considering shared or communal spaces. Although they identify personalization as a component of how spaces should be designed, the variation in how each person processes sensory information may be a barrier to doing this on a larger scale. A practical starting point in implementing dementia-friendly design in individualized client spaces is obtaining insight into the individual's sensory needs, which is discussed below in the section 'Considerations for assessment and intervention'.

A sensory lens on memory and reminiscence therapy

Reminiscence therapy is widely used with individuals with dementia, and is recommended for those with mild to moderate dementia (NICE, 2018). A variety of resources are used to support this activity, including news stories from the past, music and pictures, but the greatest gains are perhaps to be had through enhancing the sensory properties of this activity. As mentioned above, our sense of smell in particular has a strong connection with our memory and emotions and therefore may be the most effective way to support reminiscence. When encouraging recall of particular events, consider what sensory elements can be used to support recall of the experience. If discussing a particular activity perhaps consider how you can add in smells or sounds to bring the experience more to life for the individual or group, or ask the participants to recall what the sights, sounds and smells were that they encountered. Another way to facilitate this can be to introduce a certain aroma and discuss with participants what memories it naturally evokes. Using certain flavours or sweets can be another way to do this. Engaging more of our senses increases the level of stimulation and will thereby have greater cognitive benefits as part of the reminiscence.

However, while sensory input can be used to facilitate positive recall of previous life experiences, we must remember that our brains often respond to sensory cues within our environments and initiate a response before we are even aware this is occurring, particularly in response to heightened or negative memories that may have led to a fight or flight response. As a result, traumatic memories can be more easily triggered by sensory cues, indicating the importance of engaging in client-led care as part of our approach to intervention. Clients may not be able to verbally explain their negative reaction, particularly if their language skills have been compromised as a component of their dementia diagnosis, but in order to promote regulation, client-led practice and positive therapeutic rapport, quick removal of noxious sources of sensory stimulation is recommended. This will require observation of the client's responses when introducing sensory stimuli, as the person may not have the capacity to request the source of distress be removed.

Considerations for assessment and intervention

As with any client group, the best starting point for the use of sensory approaches with individuals with dementia is a comprehensive sensory assessment to identify sensory needs and responses, and how these areas impact on meaningful occupations for that person. In order to achieve such personalization in approach, a familiarity with the sensory patterns of each individual should be obtained through the use of suitable assessment resources. When choosing a means of assessment it is likely to be important to consider a balance between self-report, carer report and observations due to the impact of dementia on areas such as cognitive decline and communication.

Carer and family involvement

Depending on the level of cognitive decline, when working with individuals with dementia an increased reliance on carer report may be needed to support verification of reporting, but also to ascertain the potential impact of different environments. An individual's sensory responses observed within a clinic or care home setting are likely to differ from those in familiar environments such as their own home or different places within the community.

While the client remains the focus of the assessment and intervention phases of treatment, they may not be able to engage with the assessment process or to implement intervention strategies independently. For this reason, it is important to gain an understanding of the supports available to the person, and to identify who, if anyone, can provide meaningful information regarding your client's sensory processing. Family members, close friends, carers and healthcare staff may be included in the list of identified supports. Carer involvement may vary depending on the support needs of each client, from including others in devising the sensory plan of care, providing verbal prompts for appropriate strategy use and co-engagement using identified strategies to providing direct support for the client to access their individualized strategies.

Involvement of carers also empowers them to support the client through increased understanding of the underlying challenges and the strategies identified to assist the client to participate in their valued occupations. In living environments that have a number of staff groups (e.g. long-term care), it may be beneficial to the client to provide resources that can be used across staff groups to support implementation of the identified plan. Staff training may be a consideration, where appropriate, to increase their understanding of how sensory processing changes may present, particularly when a client has a diagnosis of dementia. Provision of education may promote the confidence of family members, carers and staff to identify potential sensory challenges and make appropriate adaptations in response to this.

There are currently limited assessments for adults that allow for both self-report and carer report in tandem. One assessment that is both validated for a sufficient age range and has both self-report and observer versions available is the Sensory Processing Measure, Second Edition (SPM-2) (Parham et al., 2021) adult form, which is norm-referenced up to 84 years of age and contains forms relating to different settings which could allow for comparison and consideration of the impact of different environments. Another assessment that may meet this need is the Adult/Adolescent Sensory History (May-Benson, 2015), which is norm-referenced for adults 13–95 years old and has both a self-report and carer report version that consider the same areas and therefore allow for comparison. There is also a medical history form that can be used alongside these and may aid consideration of the impact of other health factors on observed presentation and any pre-existing sensory and motor difficulties prior to the onset of dementia.

The Adolescent/Adult Sensory Profile (Brown & Dunn, 2002) is identified as being suitable for anyone 11 years old and up and, while it does not state an overall age range, has been informed by standardization using adults up to 97 years old (Pearson Education, 2019). The main potential limitations of this assessment for an individual with dementia are the impact of deteriorating cognition on recall and the lack of a carer report version to help confirm the results obtained. The AASP also only assesses for differences in sensory modulation, which, while an apparent need for this client group, is not the only potential need that has been suggested, and therefore it may need to be complemented with additional assessment of discrimination and praxis should these be potential concerns. An assessment that could be used to support this is Observations Based on Sensory Integration Theory (Blanche, 2010), but a number of alterations may need to be made in view of the physical limitations for this client group as well as cognitive decline. As these difficulties could apply to other client groups considered within this book, ideas for how to adapt these are provided within Chapter 8, Assessment and Goal Setting.

Approaches to intervention

Sensory-based interventions, particularly multi-sensory environments, have received ongoing attention within the literature relating to individuals with dementia, suggesting frequent use. However, there are also suggestions of a need for increased evidence of the effectiveness of sensory-based interventions with this client group, and increased staff training to support successful delivery of these interventions (Jakob & Collier, 2017). NICE (2018) guidance for dementia recommends multi-sensory stimulation for those with moderate to severe dementia, therefore it is important to consider how to gain the most benefit from sensory-based environments and activities for this client group. When used well, sensory-based interventions can be used to support meaningful engagement, reduce sensory deprivation and lessen the need for pharmacological interventions (Dimitriou et al., 2022). The benefits of access to various types of stimulation when creating a dementia-specific care package are well noted (Hughes et al., 2023; Karssemeijer et al., 2019; Strøm et al., 2016).

When using sensory approaches with this client group the primary focus is likely to be on introducing individualized strategies to reduce distress by supporting regulation, sensory-informed group activities, or environmental adaptations, which might include the use of multi-sensory environments (MSEs). All individuals with dementia are likely to benefit from sensory approaches to support regulation, even if they have no specific identified sensory needs, as they provide a low-demand way to support self-regulation. A challenge specific to this client group is likely to be that it is more difficult to obtain higher levels of certain key regulating sensory inputs such as proprioception and vestibular input due to factors such as reduced mobility, muscle weakness and comorbid physical health complaints. This may increase reliance on other regulating inputs such as deep pressure touch, and more passive vestibular input to balance obtaining regulating inputs with risk management. That is not to say that an older adult with dementia may not have difficulties with praxis or motor skills, but that there are more likely to be limitations in how much these difficulties can be assessed reliably from a sensory integration perspective.

Strategies and approaches
Sensory support plans and sensory diet

A sensory support plan or sensory diet can be an effective way to provide sensory supports throughout someone's routine or day, along with guidance for either the person themselves or others such as carers as to how and when to use certain strategies. A plan should include strategies designed both to increase and decrease levels of arousal depending on need, and the mix of such strategies is likely to look different for each individual. For further general guidance relating to sensory plans see Chapter 10, Sensory Strategies. The support required by others may vary depending on the level of cognitive impairment and stage of dementia, therefore it is helpful to provide guidance suitable for both the person themselves and those that support them. Strategies should be regularly reviewed, with an additional review following noted periods of further deterioration.

Strategies to decrease arousal

The below strategies are separated into the different sensory inputs.

VESTIBULAR AND PROPRIOCEPTIVE STRATEGIES

- Yoga or tai chi poses with adjustable levels of muscle stretch.
- Cooking or baking activities that involve kneading such as making bread or pizza dough can provide calming proprioception.
- Using a gliding chair or garden swing where available.
- Supporting engagement in activities such as walking.
- Drinking using a straw can increase proprioceptive input in the jaw and assist with regulation, alongside the tactile elements of drinking liquids.

TASTE AND OLFACTORY STRATEGIES

- Smelling aromatherapy oils such as lavender or vanilla tend to be calming for most people.
    - However, keep in mind that response to smell can also be highly individual due to the strong connection with memories, and smells that are commonly found to be alerting for some may be calming for others.

- Using scented products is an effective way to make regulating smells part of a routine and reduce the demands of initiating a strategy. Once a calming scent has been identified consider obtaining products such as shower gel or body wash with that scent.

- Eating boiled sweets can provide regulating oral-motor input.

- Drinking warm milky drinks provides calming gustatory and tactile input.

- Camomile tea calms through both gustatory and olfactory input.

- Engagement in baking or cooking activities that produce certain smells, such as baking bread or a cake, can be another way to support provision of regulating inputs.

TACTILE STRATEGIES

- Using weighted items such as a weighted cushion, weighted shawl or weighted animal.
    - Weighted items must be able to be easily removed by the client and should not be used as a form of restraint.
    - They should be used in dosed periods (i.e. considering the frequency and duration of use as a component of the recommendation).

- Using a hot water bottle or heated wheat bag.
    - Be cautious not to overheat, as tactile discrimination skills may be reduced and the client may not recognize feelings of injury due to increased temperature.
    - Electronic hot 'water' bottles are a useful substitute, as they limit the risk of burning or bursting during use.

- Altering the temperature of drinks can influence the level of arousal.

- Different thickness of drinks can add variety and increasing levels of difficulty from a proprioceptive perspective, where a risk assessment does not indicate challenges with swallowing.

- Hand massage or using massage balls allows the individual to control the amount of input and adjust it according to preference.

- Provision of a textured cushion with different elements such as buttons or varying materials.

- Wrapping a blanket around the shoulders.
    - For extra weight, this can be a wet towel applied when in the bath.
    - Consider the degree of 'stretch' of the fabric if encouraging the client to 'self-hug' using the blanket. Towelling material can be a more robust choice as it does not have the same degree of stretch as most blankets.

- Gardening activities such as potting plants.

- Using fiddle mats or cuffs. These are sleeves that can have different textures by introducing wool, buttons or other additions.

- Using a vibration cushion provides an alternative form of tactile input, which can be regulating.

- Using an electric toothbrush can be another way to introduce calming input into the day as part of a routine.

VISUAL STRATEGIES

- Provide ways to vary the level of lighting, such as a dimmer switch, lamps, fibre optic lamp or a night light.
- Pictures of preferred places, art works, family members and important events can be placed on walls or in an easily accessible place such as a box of keepsakes.
- Add colour or variation to the environment through features such as cushions or blankets to increase opportunity for clear identification of spaces and items in their environment.

AUDITORY STRATEGIES

- Playing preferred music. Generally music with a steady pace is calming, but this can vary according to preference.
- Using white noise can help to block out other distracting or problematic noises.
- Advising family members and carers not to all speak at once if in a group to prevent auditory overload.
- Taking a 'sensory break' by moving to a quieter environment temporarily – with the goal to return to a more challenging environment once the level of arousal has regulated.

Strategies to increase arousal

VESTIBULAR AND PROPRIOCEPTIVE STRATEGIES

- Dancing to familiar preferred music.
- Doing activities that involve movement of the hands such as knitting or crochet.
- Gardening activities such as watering or potting plants can help encourage movement.

TASTE AND OLFACTORY STRATEGIES

- Sucking on strong mints, or peppermint-flavoured or aniseed sweets.
- Eating citrus fruits.
- Drinking an icy/cold drink.
- Drinking mint or ginger teas.
- Smelling aromatherapy oils or scented products such as peppermint, eucalyptus and citrus scents tends to be alerting.
- Similar to the calming strategies, once a helpful scent is identified this could then be incorporated into products used at certain times of day when needing to increase alertness.

TACTILE STRATEGIES

- Having a shower set to a cooler temperature is more alerting.
  - However, when using this strategy, you should risk assess for potential factors that may make this unadvisable such as reduced temperature awareness.
  - Care should also be taken not to lower the temperature too significantly, which could potentially cause shock.
- Drinking cold or iced drinks.
- Providing smooth or textured stones or shells can provide more alerting textures.
- Running hands through dried materials such as rice.

VISUAL STRATEGIES

- Having bright or LED lighting.
- Using materials that catch and reflect light in variable ways such as mirrored material, or transparent coloured plastic or acetate sheets.
- Placing different reflective materials in shared spaces such as gardens to catch the light.
- Completing puzzles or crosswords can be visually alerting.

AUDITORY STRATEGIES

- Listening to faster-paced music or music with an irregular beat.
- Listening to music from a specific time or era to encourage memories.
- Hanging wind chimes.

Multi-sensory environments

Multi-sensory environments (MSEs) have had mixed results reported in research studies, but that is not to say they are not effective for this client group when implemented in a way that considers age appropriateness of strategies and fixtures and the ability to alter and adapt the room for the individual. Jakob and Collier produced a freely available guidebook (Jakob & Collier, 2014) to support the development of such spaces that is informed by the results of their ethnographic study evaluating spaces within 16 care homes in 2013 (Jakob & Collier, 2017). They highlight the limitations that can be common within MSEs such as giving consideration to only two or three senses and mimicking spaces designed for very different client groups that may inadvertently be over-stimulating and negatively impact arousal levels. A particular recommendation from their study is the use of different textiles and materials to provide increased levels of stimulation as well as potential for self-soothing, for example cushions with multiple textural elements and blankets that an individual can wrap around themselves to obtain deep pressure (Jakob & Collier, 2017). Their guidebook (Jakob & Collier, 2014) is freely available for individual use to support best practice in the use of MSEs.[1]

Remember that MSEs don't have to be in the form of a sensory room and could be provided in different ways to also support engagement in valued interests, such as through a sensory garden space for example. When planning these kind of areas consider providing opportunities for engagement of all the senses, ways for the individual using the space to increase or decrease the different sensory elements according to preference, and to allow them to engage in a sensory-rich routine that aims to meet their needs throughout their day.

Strategies for supporting communication

The accompanying sensory loss that is often experienced alongside the progression of dementia can further add to feelings of confusion and distress, placing increased importance on identifying supportive methods of communication and engagement. As described by Chung (2006), older adults are more likely to experience difficulty with unrelated sensory stimuli, increasing the level of challenge in maintaining focus on a conversation or task. Therefore providing grounding strategies or enhancing sensory cues that facilitate increased focus are likely to be beneficial. Below are some ways to support this:

- When providing important information, as much as possible, do so in

---

[1] Accessible at https://assets.kingston.ac.uk/m/8239cb81e12f2cb/original/How-to-make-a-Sensory-Room-for-people-with-dementia.pdf

a quiet space with reduced visual distractions to support maintenance of focus.
- Consider tone of voice and ensure it is clear and level.
- When providing written information be careful to avoid overloading a page.
- Providing a grounding tool such as a fidget item or pebble may help an individual to feel more present and sustain engagement in the conversation.

Strategies for supporting personal care

In many instances changes to the meaning and experience of personal care tasks may result in alterations to behaviour for clients with a diagnosis of dementia. Personal care is a multi-sensory activity, and in most instances places significant demand on processing tactile and proprioceptive information. Tactile processing challenges can be a source of distress as unexpected input may be perceived as an invasion of their personal space. As a result of this, it is common for clients to experience difficulties completing or allowing assistance for personal care activities, particularly as their illness progresses (Champagne, 2018). For clients with alterations to sensory processing, personal care tasks that had previously been familiar and possibly enjoyable may now be perceived as frightening. Alterations to their neurological thresholds, such as low registration of sensory information, can lead to increased levels of arousal, activation of the sympathetic nervous system responses and signs of increased anxiety or aggression. Supporting family members and carers to understand this increases their capacity to alter their approach and to incorporate strategies which work for the client.

These ideas may include:

- Approaching the client from the front only. This will promote feelings of safety as they can visually identify who is approaching them as well as assisting with identifying proximity to others in their environment.

- Clearly indicating who you are and why you are there. This may be repeated, if necessary, throughout the encounter.

- If touching to assist with transfer, positioning or self-care is required, verbally identifying what you are going to do before doing it is important.
  - Give them time to process this information (e.g. 'Mary, I am going to put my hand on your arm'). When you have placed your hand,

identify that it is your hand and continue to clearly state what will happen next.

- Using firm, open palm touch only when assisting with self-care tasks.
    - Light touch has been shown to be activating and can be experienced by many clients as an unsafe form of tactile input.
- Encouraging the client to assist with or complete the task where possible will allow them to have a level of control over the level of sensory stimulation they are receiving.
- Reducing the pace of the task when moving through the steps allows for extra time, which is useful for clients to process what is happening as delayed nerve conductivity is a feature of the ageing process.
- Providing choices on what tools are used allows for the inclusion of their sensory preferences (e.g. a loofah versus a sponge).
- Ask the client to 'test' water prior to supporting them into a bath or under a shower to ensure their experience of the temperature is comfortable.
- If using scented bathing products, ensure the client has identified the scent as enjoyable.
    - Noxious olfactory information can directly impact emotional regulation and may contribute to distress.
- Minimize unnecessary sources of environmental stimulation, such as background noise, where possible to reduce the likelihood of overwhelm.
- Consider any previous trauma history, and how this impacts on how personal care should be managed (e.g. clients who have experienced trauma may require personal care to be carried out by same-gender staff members).

CASE STUDY – Dana
Background
Dana, 72 years old, was referred to occupational therapy services by her consultant psychiatrist following an outpatient appointment for assessment of functioning and work on social engagement. She was noted to have a diagnosis of mixed dementia (vascular and Alzheimer's types), and was experiencing signs of agitation, anxiety and social isolation. She lived with her husband and had three adult children. They identified that she seemed particularly anxious and distressed when the family called to see her.

Assessment and formulation of difficulties
Assessments completed included the Occupational Self-Assessment (Baron et al., 2006), Adolescent/Adult Sensory Profile (Brown & Dunn, 2002), Sensory Processing Caregiver Checklist (Champagne, 2018) completed by Dana's husband and children, and clinical observations of sensory integration. Results of the assessments suggested difficulties with tactile and vestibular discrimination (subjectively reported) and proprioceptive discrimination (objectively and subjectively reported). Dana experienced heightened sensitivity to auditory input and low registration for movement, tactile and olfactory input.

A hypothesis was developed that Dana had challenges with proprioceptive discrimination, which negatively influenced her confidence and ability to engage socially, thus contributing to self-isolation. Dana's difficulties modulating sensory information, specifically under-responsivity to proprioceptive, vestibular and tactile stimulation, and over-responsivity to auditory stimulation, were impacting on her ability to tolerate social situations.

Intervention
Intervention focused on regulation of arousal levels to help improve tolerance for social situations through development of strategies to form part of her daily routine. This included the use of deep pressure touch strategies such as wrapping a blanket around her shoulders and use of an electric hot water bottle, and movement opportunities such as going for a walk and trialling yoga. To support management of auditory input, strategies were implemented such as family encouraging Dana to take a break from social gatherings as needed and being mindful to not all speak at once. Use of preferred music was also encouraged for regulation. In addition to this, psychoeducation was provided to Dana's family to help them recognize

signs of becoming overwhelmed due to her challenges modulating auditory information, and to identify and offer appropriate management strategies.

CONCLUSION/KEY LEARNING

This chapter considers the evidence in relation to sensory processing changes that may be experienced in connection with dementia but also as part of the natural ageing process. Consideration should be given to how this might inform the support provided to an individual with dementia and facilitate a reduction in the behavioural and psychological symptoms of dementia.

Key points

- Sensory changes are a naturally occurring part of the age process but may increase the levels of agitation experienced for someone with dementia.
- Reframing behaviours from a sensory perspective can inform more tailored individualized support and enable positive engagement.
- Carers and family members are an integral part of the assessment and intervention process with this client group.

CHAPTER 8

Assessment and Goal Setting

LEANNE DUGGAN AND REBECCA MATSON

Choosing a suitable assessment is invaluable in all areas of occupational therapy, and doing so when identifying an individual's sensory needs is no exception to this. Everyone has sensory needs and everyone can benefit from using sensory approaches, but completion of a screening tool or assessment allows for a more targeted intervention and greater intentionality in the use of strategies. Completion of a thorough assessment also supports a more comprehensive consideration of an individual's sensory processing challenges, and their impacts upon functioning.

Attention within mental health is often given to sensory modulation, which, while incredibly important, does not encompass the full extent of possible sensory processing difficulties. Champagne et al. (2010) discuss how sensory discrimination issues often co-occur with modulation difficulties in mental health but can be missed, or are assumed to relate to hypo- or hyper-responsivity to sensory input. The risk of this error increases when assumptions are made on the basis of how someone presents in the absence of a comprehensive assessment. An inadequate understanding of the specific nature of the difficulty could lead to an ineffective intervention approach and continued feelings of confusion for that individual. In addition to this, praxis difficulties are also prevalent amongst those with mental health conditions and can be a significant cause of frustration and provide added barriers to independent functioning and engagement in valued activities.

A sensory assessment is an important part of understanding our clients but also of supporting them to understand their own needs and develop strategies for self-management. The explanation of the results of a sensory assessment is often the first step in intervention and can put together the pieces in relation to difficulties an individual has been experiencing for years without knowing why, and while experiencing judgement from others who make assumptions about the reason for their difficulties.

Identifying an appropriate sensory assessment tool

While overall there is a relative lack of sensory assessments that are standardized for use with adult populations, this is improving and there are now a few comprehensive self-report assessments that can be used, such as:

- the Adolescent/Adult Sensory Profile (AASP) (Brown & Dunn, 2002)
- the Adult/Adolescent Sensory History (ASH) (May-Benson, 2015)
- the Sensory Processing Measure, Second Edition (SPM-2) (Parham et al., 2021).

All of the above are validated to cover a broad age range including older adults. The information contained within this chapter will help you to consider when each may be most suitable. Table 8.1 provides an overview of the main criteria in relation to a number of these assessments and appears at the end of this chapter for ease of reference.

There remains a lack of performance-based assessments to more comprehensively assess sensory processing in the context of praxis and motor skills. The Sensory Processing 3-Dimensions Scale (SP3D) (Miller, Schoen & Mulligan, date of publication pending), which at the time of writing is undergoing establishment of norms for various age ranges including adults, will provide an assessment to meet this gap. In the interim, assessments such as the Sensory Integration and Praxis Test (SIPT) (Ayres, 1989) and its successor, the Evaluation in Ayres Sensory Integration (EASI), are used with adults, but with caution, and as yet do not provide any norms for adults. As these assessments take a developmental perspective it could be assumed that an adult should be able to achieve the higher end of the age norms, but there are added complicating factors to consider such as sensory decline with age, and the impact of comorbid conditions.

However, in the absence as yet of a fully suitable assessment, consideration will be given below to how the SIPT, the EASI and the Structured Observations of Sensory Integration – Motor (SOSI-M) (Blanche et al., 2021) could be cautiously used with adult client groups. Ayres Clinical Observations (Blanche et al., 2020) will also be discussed as a non-standardized option for gaining greater insight, as well as the Assessment of Motor and Process Skills (AMPS) (Fisher, 2006, 2010), which while not a sensory assessment is standardized for adults and provides relevant assessment data to inform a sensory assessment. Consideration will also be given to informal clinical observations and how an individual's sensory processing needs could be assessed during commonly administered functional assessments used within occupational therapy practice.

Individuals who are under adult mental health services often undergo a high number of different assessments and therefore it may not be possible or reasonable to carry out as many assessments as is ideal. However, much information can be gathered from observing everyday activities to inform a sensory assessment, therefore ideas for this will also be considered within this chapter. This fits well with the overarching perspective of sensory integration theory, as assessment is only necessary if there are identified participation challenges, which will be experienced within the context of the client's daily activities.

Self-report and carer report assessments
Adolescent/Adult Sensory Profile (AASP) (Brown & Dunn, 2002)

The AASP is the most well established of the assessments for adults and also the most researched, with it being the most frequently used choice for studies identifying the sensory processing patterns of different diagnostic groups. Studies have been completed in relation to individuals with:

- schizophrenia
- OCD
- depression and anxiety
- bipolar disorder
- PTSD
- dementia.

(Brown et al., 2002; Halperin & Falk-Kessler, 2020; Rieke & Anderson, 2009; Serafini et al., 2016; Zhou et al., 2020)

This can make it a good choice if you are trying to establish the prevalence of sensory needs amongst your client group, and it is important to be able to compare your results to the outcomes of published studies, for example if attempting to secure funding for resources.

The assessment follows Dunn's (1997) model of sensory processing, which categorizes responses according to neurological threshold and behavioural responses. It identifies four categories within this:

- Low registration

- This relates to someone with a high threshold for sensory input and who demonstrates a passive response to it; that is, they need a high amount of sensory input to notice it but do not actively try to meet that threshold.

- Sensation seeking
  - Sensation seeking also relates to someone with a high threshold for sensory input, but with an active response; they actively find ways to gain the additional sensory input they need.

- Sensory sensitivity
  - Sensory sensitivity relates to a low threshold but with a passive response – someone who becomes easily overwhelmed by sensory input but does not tend to implement active strategies to reduce it.

- Sensory avoiding
  - Sensory avoiding also relates to a low threshold, but with an active response; in contrast to someone who is sensory sensitive, they would actively find ways to minimize the sensory input and to manage it.

The AASP provides results in relation to each of these categories as to how strong an influence that pattern has on a person.

PROS OF THE AASP

Overall, strong patterns have been seen using the AASP with different groups, and it is helpful in highlighting the impact of sensory processing on an individual's day-to-day presentation, particularly in relation to their levels of regulation. The results of individual studies are discussed further in the diagnosis-specific chapters. The results of the assessment are relatively easy to explain to someone and relate well to terms commonly used within mental health services. The AASP has been suggested as having good discriminative validity (Brown et al., 2002; Engel-Yeger et al., 2013) and good internal consistency, with coefficient alpha values for the adult age group ranging from 0.639 to 0.699 for each of the subscales (Brown & Dunn, 2002).

CONS OF THE AASP

The main limitation of the AASP is that it only assesses modulation and therefore on its own cannot be called a comprehensive assessment of sensory processing. The results are also not broken down into the different sensory systems, which is an important consideration in identifying how someone's reactions may vary according to the different inputs. Individuals can often fall into different categories in relation to the different senses, therefore this is important to consider to inform intervention approaches, and ensure they are specific to individual need. This therefore places additional demands on the therapist in reviewing answers to individual questions to inform more specific hypotheses of need. The scoring page of the AASP does list the results for each question within a category in clusters of the different senses, so it can be relatively easy to identify areas of high scores in connection with a particular sense, but as there are no norms for the individual senses it leaves identifying what is significant much more to individual therapist judgement (Blanche et al., 2014). The assessment also only includes a self-report version, which may be a limitation when working with certain client groups where there is a need to gather additional perspectives or to complete the assessment through a proxy.

There are a number of questions within this assessment where an element of caution may be needed in interpreting the responses, due to the potential for these to be impacted by other factors. Therefore, it is especially important once overall scoring has been completed to return to the questions and identify those that have influenced the score in a particular area to 'sense-check' and consider if the results are congruent with daily experience and presentation. For example, questions about becoming dizzy easily or only eating familiar foods are highly likely to be impacted by other factors for someone with an eating disorder and low dietary intake. Similarly, layering of clothing or wearing long sleeves and trousers regardless of weather can also be intended to prevent others from seeing their body shape and weight. Or an individual with OCD may avoid crowds or move away when others get too close due to fear of germs rather than a difficulty with tolerating tactile input. This again calls on therapist judgement to decipher where this may have been the case and to revisit those areas with the client.

Adult/Adolescent Sensory History (ASH) (May-Benson, 2015)
The ASH is a much more recently available assessment for adults, and while as yet it does not have the same level of established research it is becoming widely accepted and used within mental health settings, primarily due to an increased comprehensiveness that covers sensory modulation, discrimination, praxis, postural control, motor skills and gravitational insecurity. It has been validated for the adult population and has been found effective in identifying differences between a normative population and those with sensory processing

disorders (May-Benson, 2015). Concurrent validity was established through comparison with the AASP, finding a significant level of correlation ($r = 0.78$, $p < 0.001$) (Barker et al., 2015), and there is also a high level of test–retest reliability (Pearson's r values between 0.74 and 0.88) (May-Benson, 2015). The age range covered extends from 13 to 95 years old.

The ASH has self-report, caregiver report, an abridged self-report version and a medical questionnaire (May-Benson, 2015). Caution is recommended when using the caregiver report version as a study comparing the ratings of adults themselves and those completed by parents found that parents tended to be more prone to under-reporting (May-Benson & Easterbrooks-Dick, 2016). Therefore, wherever possible it is advisable to also obtain some form of self-report to supplement this version.

PROS OF THE ASSESSMENT

The assessment is accompanied with scoring software that produces a report providing z scores for each of the senses in relation to modulation and discrimination, different aspects of motor coordination, postural control, gravitational insecurity and social emotional factors, and overall scores for each of the sensory systems. Based upon the scores, each area is rated as either typical, mild difficulty or severe difficulty, guiding the clinician as to the primary areas of concern. The manual also provides detail of the specific questions that influence the different overall scores, allowing the therapist to see which areas had the biggest impact and check back with the person as needed to identify any potential red herrings.

CONS OF THE ASSESSMENT

While the ASH reduces therapist burden in relation to analysis, it does require a certain level of knowledge and understanding in the therapist to consider the results of the assessment as a comprehensive whole and to use the results to guide a suitable intervention. However, the assessment overall is quick to administer and provides a detailed overview of sensory processing needs to guide a therapist's hypothesis and identify the need for any further assessment in relation to areas such as motor skills.

Similar to the AASP, there may be questions where the answers could be impacted by other factors, and again it would be advisable to check through the questions that have incurred a high score on a certain area. Pages 21–22 in the manual (May-Benson, 2015) support you in doing this by clustering the questions that have informed certain section scores. Where there is considered to be a higher risk of this occurring it may be useful to complete the medical supplement available with this assessment to gather supporting information. In this case it would also be advisable to either complete the assessment in person with the individual or go back to them for more information about certain questions afterwards to gain further information.

Sensory Processing Measure, Second Edition (SPM-2)

While the original Sensory Processing Measure (Parham & Ecker, 2007) has been in use in a variety of settings, a version standardized for adults has only been available since 2021. The assessment has self-report and carer forms as well as a driving form, to assess whether sensory processing issues might impact an individual's ability to drive safely, with the adult forms being suitable for ages 21–87. The results provide scores in relation to processing of visual, auditory, tactile, olfactory, gustatory, proprioceptive and vestibular input as well as praxis and social participation, identifying each area as being of 'no difference', 'probable difference' or 'definite difference'. A report is produced that suggests the level of difficulty expected based upon the scores in different sections; for example, a high score would suggest difficulties across both modulation and praxis to co-exist.

PROS OF THE ASSESSMENT

The availability of both self-report and carer report versions of the assessment form is of benefit where there is a need to gain and integrate both perspectives. The online scoring system increases the ease of comparisons between forms completed by the individual and a carer or between two different carers or raters. There is also the option to use a paper form or send a direct link to the assessment form for the individual to complete that is then automatically scored by the online system, easing overall demand on the therapist. The SPM-2 has high levels of internal consistency for the sensory total score (0.90) and test–retest reliability. Similar to the ASH, the levels of inter-rater reliability are only moderate, but this is thought to be due to factors such as observing the individual in different contexts (0.78 for sensory total score).

CONS OF THE ASSESSMENT

While the report generates scores for each of the senses, the results of the different senses are not separated into areas of difficulty such as modulation and discrimination. This therefore requires the therapist to examine individual questions to fully identify the specific nature of the difficulty. Similar to the ASH, therefore, this requires an increased level of knowledge on the part of the therapist, but the manual also has a section where each of the questions is connected to the area they assess within that sense. For example, each question in the visual section is either linked to over-reactivity, under-reactivity, perception of sensory input or ocular-motor skills.

Assessing interoception

Interoception is a growing field within sensory integration theory. Identifying potential interoceptive challenges as part of your assessment when generating a hypothesis involves identifying and evaluating how the person experiences their internal sensations. Interoceptive functioning impacts on a number of areas, including emotional processing and sleep (Birba et al., 2022; Hazelton et al., 2023; Mahler, 2017; Salamone et al., 2021; Wei & Van Someren, 2020). These are significant considerations within mental health practice, and the ability of the person to perceive and tolerate their internal experiences is a concern relevant to sensory processing assessment as it allows for further analysis of how the person perceives and uses sensation as a component of their everyday functioning.

Assessment resources

For many, this may be an unfamiliar area of assessment. Using a checklist such as the Multidimensional Assessment of Interoceptive Awareness, Version 2 (MAIA-2) may be a good starting point. This was developed by the University of California, San Francisco, and is available within the public domain (Mehling et al., 2018).[1] This checklist can be used to provide a framework around which discussions about interoceptive experiences can be framed, but is reliant on the client being able to engage in the self-rating system at a meaningful level to fully identify potential challenges. This information can be used in conjunction with other sensory assessments as a component of your formulation to give further insight into the client's internal sensory world.

An additional component of the AASP, the Sensory Processing Interoception (SPI) scale, is due to become available and focuses on assessment of interoception, which will provide another option for assessment. Similar to the focus of the AASP itself, the measure will assess interoception in the context of participation, with a particular focus on self-care, eating and completion of an individual's daily routine (Dunn et al., 2022). The items of the scale have been found to have good internal consistency and a high level of correlation with the items on the AASP itself. The focus on measurement through experience of

---

1   Accessible at https://osher.ucsf.edu/research/maia

daily activities may make this measure more accessible to those who experience alexithymia and struggle to describe their internal experiences as it may provide something more tangible to consider when responding to the questions.

Non-standardized sensory screening tools

In addition to the above more formal assessments, there are a range of screening tools available if your initial aim is to gain further understanding of an individual's sensory preferences in general. Tina Champagne has a freely available sensory diet checklist, similar to an interest checklist, on her website OT-Innovations that could help gain an idea of strategies an individual may wish to try.[2] She has also included a carer sensory checklist in her book *Sensory Modulation in Dementia Care* (Champagne, 2018), which is useful where additional information is available from family or carers. This may assist with establishing further information to help identify an overall pattern of sensory integration dysfunction. Sensory Modulation Brisbane also have a Sensory Preferences Screen, focused on considering the office environment, and a Sensory Triggers Screen, focused on a medical ward environment.[3] While these tools will not provide you with a comprehensive assessment they could be a helpful starting point in discussing sensory needs with someone and less demanding than a formal assessment measure.

Performance-based assessments

Currently there are no performance-based assessments for adults that measure sensory motor functions comprehensively. Therefore, while not validated for this purpose, a number of therapists utilize assessments validated for child age ranges to support the assessment process. Overall, these assessments are based upon developmental stages, so an adult could be expected to perform at the higher end of the scoring, but much caution is needed as there are also a range of additional factors to consider that complicate the picture, such as the development of splinter skills that may mask the level of actual difficulty and age-related sensory loss or deterioration. These assessments are therefore generally used in a more informal way to gain additional information through observations rather than application of standardized scores. Champagne and Koomar (2012) offer support for this approach to assessment, suggesting that

---

2   Available at www.ot-innovations.com/wp-content/uploads/2013/09/sensory_diet_checklist_2007pdf.pdf
3   Available at sensory-modulation-brisbane.com

if a certain level of skills is expected of a child, this should be fully developed in the adult population. However, they advise caution as the test can then no longer be considered standardized and becomes simply a way of gathering clinical observations.

Evaluation in Ayres Sensory Integration (EASI) (Mailloux, et al., 2018)

The EASI forms an updated version of the SIPT, with assessment of the additional areas of sensory reactivity and sensory perception to provide a more comprehensive overall assessment. The assessment is designed to be more readily accessible and affordable than its predecessor, as the therapist builds much of the kit from more readily available items, and once the relevant training has been completed a therapist has free access to the scoring software for a year. Rather than a pay per assessment system, the EASI has a set annual fee to retain access to the scoring programme.

The EASI takes approximately 1.5–2 hours to administer, therefore may need to be completed over multiple sessions depending on the person and their individual needs. As the assessment is designed to engage a child, a potential barrier is the format of certain sub-tests, which use language or activities intended for younger populations. Use of the EASI also requires you to have completed a certain level of sensory integration training (specific level is dependent on the training provider) and demands a good level of understanding to accurately interpret the results.

Currently, however, the EASI is only standardized for children between the ages of 3 and 12 years old and is not validated for adults. Therefore caution would be recommended in use with adults. However, there is the potential for useful qualitative information and insight into an individual's sensory processing and responses that could be gained through selection of relevant sub-tests to support other forms of assessment or where there is a gap in the assessment data that has been obtained.

Sensory Integration and Praxis Test (SIPT) (Ayres, 1989)

The SIPT had been considered the 'gold standard' for sensory integration assessment prior to the release of the EASI, which builds on the foundations set by this assessment. It contains 17 tests that measure sensory integration and praxis, including tactile processing, vestibular-proprioceptive processing, visual perception and praxis. The SIPT has strong inter-rater reliability ranging between 0.94 and 0.99, but reliability is lower when interpreting the scores in relation to specific patterns of sensory processing disorder (Asher et al., 2008).

Discriminative validity was established with a sample of 239 typically developing children and children with disabilities, in which all of the tests discriminated between the two groups at $p < 0.01$ (Ayres, 2004). However, as the SIPT is only standardized on children between the ages of 4 years and 8 years 11 months, its potential application to an adult client group is questionable (Cermak, 1992).

Research studies have established adult norms for specific sub-tests, including post-rotary nystagmus (Utley et al., 1983), and the tactile tests, many of which, while not standardized for adults, were developed out of neurological tests often used on adults, and therefore have some transferability (Hsu & Nelson, 1981). Hsu and Nelson (1981) found ceiling effects in the testing of adults from the general population, suggesting that below-average results on the tactile tests may be of significance. However, there are no more recent studies into its use with adults and caution may need to be taken in applying these norms. If using the SIPT with adult clients, it therefore may be best to utilize with caution and to base interpretation on qualitative information gained through observations rather than formal scoring.

The SIPT, however, has been said to require a high level of knowledge and skill to ensure accurate interpretation of the results, and in order to administer the assessment therapists are required to have completed a certain level of post-graduate training in sensory integration. It is also a relatively lengthy assessment, taking around two hours to complete in full. As the SIPT has been updated and expanded to form the EASI, its use is no longer taught. However, for those who have access to it, use of specific sub-tests may support further focused assessment where needed. For example, the Figure–Ground Perception (FG) test can be helpful where visual discrimination difficulties are suspected, and may help to provide further objective information in areas not covered by the clinical observations. Use with an adult mental health population should therefore be considered cautiously but not ruled out as a possibility.

Structured Observations of Sensory Integration – Motor (SOSI-M) (Blanche et al., 2021)

The SOSI-M is a standardized assessment that is designed to assess vestibular processing, proprioception, postural control and motor planning through building on Ayres Clinical Observations. Alongside it is a supporting observation tool, the Complete Observations of Proprioception (COP-R), intended to gather further information on proprioceptive processing through behavioural observations. As the assessment is standardized it has an added benefit for clinical observations in that it does provide scores for the different areas measured and remains relatively quick to administer, taking around 20–40 minutes to complete. It has strong overall internal consistency of 0.85 and inter-rater reliability of 0.98. However, it is only standardized for children aged 5–14 and is not currently validated for adults, and the authors have advised caution in using it with adults due to the complexity of the ageing process and potential confounding factors.

Sensory Processing 3-Dimensions Scale (SP3D) (Miller, Schoen & Mulligan, date of publication pending)

The SP3D is a new test of sensory processing that will enable assessment across much of the life span from three years old through to adulthood. The assessment has followed on from the Sensory Processing Scale (Schoen et al., 2014), which is focused on measurement of sensory modulation but also measures discrimination and motor-based abilities. It will expand on the areas of praxis measured by the SIPT to also consider ideational praxis, an area that has a potentially significant impact on motor skills. This will be the first sensory processing performance-based assessment to support standardized assessment across the life span.

Assessment of Motor and Process Skills (AMPS) (Fisher, 2006, 2010)

While the AMPS is not a sensory integration assessment due to the focus on motor and process skills, it can provide helpful information on these areas to complement sensory processing tools and support consideration of potentially connected praxis issues. The assessment is standardized and provides a computer-generated report that considers the impact of 16 motor skills and 20 process skills on an individual's performance in familiar, relevant activities of daily living, and potential levels of independence based upon this. Training to learn to use the AMPS assessment has been unavailable since 31 May 2023, but it is included here because those who already have training may find it a useful support in their assessment process. A particular strength of the AMPS is that it provides the individual with the opportunity to demonstrate their skill level through mirroring everyday task performance.

The AMPS report provides insight into how efficient, effortful and organized an individual's performance was, which helps to inform assessment of praxis. Information from the AMPS could therefore help to consider whether it is the ideation, planning or execution stage that is problematic when an individual is struggling with praxis. However, keep in mind that the AMPS results alone would not confirm sensory-based motor difficulties; in order to decide if the motor difficulties have a sensory basis it would be important to also assess tactile, vestibular and proprioceptive processing in particular.

Structured clinical observations

There are several versions of clinical observations available, some of which are freely accessible online. Completion of structured clinical observations has generally been recommended to complement the assessment process (Asher et al., 2008; Schaaf et al., 2014). While they are not standardized, they can provide valuable contextual information, but require greater effort and interpretation on the part of the therapist. Ayres Clinical Observations primarily focus on tests that show vestibular, proprioceptive and tactile processing but also include visual processing. Within the clinical observations the tests often completed include diadochokinesis (forearm alternating movements), supine flexion, prone extension, sequential finger touching and Schilder's Arm Extension Test alongside tests of postural control and gravitational security (Blanche et al., 2020).

Similar to the SOSI-M, Ayres Clinical Observations are relatively quick to administer and may be more accessible to adult client groups than assessments such as the SIPT or EASI as they don't include some of the aspects or structures designed to engage children that other assessments may contain. Versions such as that by Blanche (2010) contain guidance videos and supporting information on how long a child should be able to hold a position such as supine flexion, or guidance as to what may indicate effective performance. As with the SIPT, it could be assumed that an adult should be able to perform as well as the highest age range considered, but age-related comorbidities or decline that may alter performance need to be borne in mind. Further information on clinical observations that can be used and how to interpret them is available in Blanche et al. (2020), but, similar to Blanche (2010), is focused on children.

It is important for clinicians to use their clinical judgement to ascertain the necessity of completing all clinical observation tasks, or whether strategically chosen test items will allow for the formulation of a sensory hypothesis on which to build goals and a clear treatment plan. Blanche et al. (2020, p. 236) identify the importance of having 'multiple data points that indicate a deficit' when evaluating sensory processing. Multiple sources of information allow the clinician to distinguish a pattern of dysfunction from a once-off occurrence or observed behaviour which may or may not be related to the overall ability of the client to process sensory information.

Potential barriers to completing clinical observations

When working with an adult population, it may be necessary to adjust your assessment process to enable the client to engage with the assessment in a way that is safe, while still allowing for clear identification of sensory-based challenges. One barrier to completing clinical observations with adults can be factors such as age-related decline in postural control, increasing levels of frailty, deterioration in visual acuity, decreased flexibility or weight-related barriers. These clients may require alterations to the assessment process to accommodate their needs, and these can be documented as a consideration for your clinical reasoning when formulating your sensory hypothesis.

Below are ideas on how to adapt some of the clinical observations that can be more problematic:

- Gravitational security: Rather than tipping an individual backwards on a gym ball, gravitational insecurity can be assessed by observing stability when sitting on a gym ball (as this is more apparent when seated with no back) or by asking the person to sit on an office chair and tilting the upper part backwards slightly.

- Prone extension and supine flexion: These test items require the client to move to the floor as a component of assessment. For clients with mobility challenges or a fear of falling, this may not be an action that they are willing to complete. The function of these test items is to assess the ability to assume the positions indicated, rather than the ability to position themselves on a certain surface. Therefore, alterations can be made such as asking a client to perform these tasks on a raised surface, such as a bed, rather than the floor – as long as they can observe the therapist demonstrating the positions first. This can be noted as a qualitative point as a component of your observational notes, and can be considered within the overall performance of the client across test items.

Additional important assessment considerations

There are often added challenges to obtaining an accurate sensory assessment with an adult who is likely to have developed a range of splinter skills and ways to mask the impact of their sensory processing difficulties, which may need to be unpicked. In addition, there can be a number of confounding factors that complicate the picture and require careful clinical reasoning to evaluate and interpret within the context of the client's overall presentation and functioning.

While not exhaustive, the following list of factors may influence the accuracy of sensory assessments, and should be considered to support a clear identification of underlying challenges.

Symptoms of specific mental health conditions

Mental health symptoms influence how a client perceives and lives within the world and could potentially alter their responses during sensory assessments. It is not possible to list all possible such factors here, but an example of this is experience of paranoia and the resultant hyper-vigilance that may occur due to a belief that they are likely to experience harm or that others intend them harm (Raihani & Bell, 2019). Therefore, when conducting a self-rated sensory assessment such as the Adult/Adolescent Sensory History (ASH), statements such as 'become distracted by lots of noise' (May-Benson, 2015, p. 3) could be interpreted in a different manner to that intended. While this statement aims to assess sensory responsivity, this difficulty could also be seen as a result of a need to constantly be aware of their environment in order to maintain their safety, rather than due to having a low neurological threshold for auditory input. Symptomology such as this is a particularly important consideration when assessing adults with mental health conditions, to evaluate whether your assessment results could be attributed to symptoms of illness rather than an underlying sensory processing challenge.

Medication side effects

Medications used to treat mental health conditions may also influence how clients process sensation. An important example of this, and one that is likely to be frequently observed in mental health settings, is the impact of antipsychotic medications on motor skills in clients with psychotic disorders. Extrapyramidal side effects (EPSEs) or drug-induced movement disorders (Ali et al., 2021) are an unwanted, adverse impact of using antipsychotics, which directly affects the client's ability to plan and execute purposeful motor activity. These can be evident in indicators such as a tremor, facial tics and muscle stiffness. A systematic review of antipsychotic-induced EPSEs by Ali et al. (2021) identified the prevalence rate of EPSEs as between 31 per cent and 37 per cent for clients prescribed antipsychotics, making this an important consideration. As part of a sensory assessment with a client who is prescribed antipsychotic medication, motor skills and praxis should still be considered, but in view of the likelihood of this being connected to their medication rather than as a component of difficulties integrating sensation. Where it is unclear if the motor difficulties observed are a result of EPSEs, gaining a developmental history could help identify if they pre-existed medication use.

Ageing and sensory loss

Sensory changes occur as a natural part of the ageing process, including alterations to the number of neurons and level of connectivity (National Institute on Ageing, 2023). These changes can impact the brain globally, and may contribute to impairment across multiple sensory systems, resulting in a significant impact on how older adults process sensation. Older adults may also experience changes in their perception of sensation, requiring the assistance of equipment such as glasses or hearing aids to promote engagement and function. Where difficulties are identified in relation to visual or auditory processing, consideration should always be given to whether a recent eye test or hearing test has taken place.

Peripheral nervous system (PNS) changes

Changes to structures within the PNS as a result of injury or the ageing process will alter how the brain perceives and processes sensation. Correia et al. (2016) (N = 2968) identified that tactile discrimination declines with age due to decreased nerve conduction velocity, decreased density of tactile receptors and grey matter changes in the central nervous system (CNS). Despite an individual presenting with a sensory processing challenge, sensory-based treatment in this case will not result in an improvement in function, as it is unlikely to influence the nerve conduction speed in the CNS. However, a sensory assessment may still be of benefit to such clients to identify specific areas of challenge in their sensory processing and the impact of this on their daily life. This can contribute to the development of a sensory-informed treatment plan that is reflective of the challenges influencing function, participation and safety within the client's everyday lives.

Changes in cognition

Changes to cognitive abilities will impact on the ability of the client to engage with the assessment process. Cognitive impairment can occur as a result of a number of mental health conditions, either as a temporary or longer-term impact. Where this is the case, splitting an assessment across a number of shorter sessions and ensuring clients have adequate time in which to understand and answer questions are useful strategies in subjectively rated assessments. In this instance, it may be necessary to work with others to gain information relating to the client's sensory processing. Useful information could be gathered from supporting staff members, carers and family. While potentially a less comprehensive assessment, this will give a perspective on how those providing care are experiencing the client, and whether there are any indications that their ability to process sensation may be a contributing factor to their level of distress. From a safety perspective, direct assessment with clients experiencing cognitive impairment should include an evaluation of the individual's ability to follow verbal and visual instructions prior to initiating clinical observations.

To reduce the impact of confounding factors on your practice, it is important to identify and incorporate them into your clinical reasoning. Central to this is identifying and using your population-specific knowledge. Features of illness, treatment approaches and diagnosis-specific presentations may all have an influence on how a client processes sensation, but this may resolve as they progress along their treatment pathway. By reflecting on how other factors influence your sensory assessment formulation, you will introduce a holistic framework on which to build when identifying the degree of a client's sensory processing challenges, and the impact they have on their ability to participate in meaningful occupations.

Gathering supporting information from others

In some instances, it may not be possible to rely solely on the assessment data obtained from the client themselves. Confounding factors such as those outlined above may influence the client's ability to engage with the assessment process and could alter the reliability of the results. Assessments can also place a significant demand on clients, which may cause distress or risk disengagement. Where participation challenges have been identified, it may therefore be appropriate to gather information from others to assist with discerning if further assessment would be beneficial and to inform the overall assessment itself. This has a number of advantages, which include:

- Gaining a perspective on a client's functioning across a broader time period and more settings than you may be able to observe.
- An opportunity to gather further information where a client is identified as having limited insight into their own functional challenges.
- Development of rapport with family members and carers, who may later be asked to assist with the implementation of intervention strategies. Completion of such assessments could also help build understanding of why intervention is needed and the purpose of chosen approaches.

Sensory-informed functional assessments and observations

While it may be ideal to have a range of sensory assessments completed as part of your assessment process, it can be difficult to achieve this without overwhelming the client, who may be undergoing other assessments within a service, or when in the earlier stages of developing rapport, for example. There is also a range of valuable information you can gain to inform assessment of sensory processing while completing functional assessments or semi-structured interviews, or when observing engagement in activities. While not an exhaustive list, the information below will help you consider some potential indicators of difficulty in different areas of sensory processing.

Areas of difficulty in sensory processing
VESTIBULAR DISCRIMINATION

- Becoming disorientated easily.
- Overbalancing when bending down to pick up something or leaning over.
- Toe walking can be a sign of vestibular discrimination (consider cautiously as there can also be other reasons).
- Propping against objects or surfaces for support during tasks that require standing for periods of time (e.g. when stirring a pot on the hob).
- Flinching away from fast-moving objects (e.g. cars travelling at speed towards them).
- Travel sickness or discomfort when they are a passenger in a car.

PROPRIOCEPTIVE DISCRIMINATION

- Closing doors heavily/accidentally slamming doors.
- Accidentally breaking items frequently.
- A need to watch their feet when walking up or down stairs.
- Holding tightly to the handrail in elevators or escalators, or when using stairs.
- Bumping into door frames.
- Being 'heavy footed' when walking.
- Using too much force when spreading toast, causing the bread to tear.
- Difficulty sustaining body position when seated and maybe slouching or propping themselves up.
- 'Wall walking', that is, touching the wall with their hand when walking to ensure they remain an adequate distance away from it.

TACTILE DISCRIMINATION

- Demonstrating a need to keep different foods separate on a plate.

- Avoidance of food choices with mixed textures/limited food choices.
- Difficulty selecting the right coin from their pocket or wallet.
- Difficulty finding an item in a bag or drawer without looking.
- Limited clothing choices and preferences, for example keeping to similar fabrics.
- Limited variety of textures within home décor.
- Difficulty identifying changes in temperature, either in the atmosphere around them or in relation to food.

VISUAL DISCRIMINATION

- Difficulty finding a specific utensil in the utensil drawer or picking out items in the fridge or cupboard from amongst others.
- Difficulty gauging when it is safe to cross the road.
- Losing their place in a recipe on a page or website.
- Difficulty finding their way around a supermarket or shop.
- Difficulty locating an item on a shelf.
- Difficulty identifying appliances amongst others in kitchen cupboards.
- Difficulty identifying when tasks have been sufficiently completed, for example mixing ingredients together sufficiently when cooking.
- Inability to tolerate clutter/becoming overwhelmed in cluttered environments.

AUDITORY DISCRIMINATION

- Asking for questions or instructions to be repeated frequently.
- Difficulty engaging in conversation in busy areas.
- Significantly delayed response times when having a conversation (n.b. it is essential to consider if the client may have any hearing challenges and when they last had their hearing checked).

INTEROCEPTIVE DISCRIMINATION

- Difficulties noticing when they need to use the bathroom until it is extremely urgent.
- Difficulties identifying when they are hungry or thirsty.
- Heightened anxiety response to internal sensations.
- Experiencing uncomfortable internal sensations (e.g. wiggling or butterflies) without an identifiable cause, leading to significant distress.

VESTIBULAR MODULATION

- Intolerance of movements of head when bending down to complete tasks.
- Avoidance of bending in certain ways, for example bending at the knees in order to keep head raised.
- Avoidance of rotational or circular movements, such as going on certain fairground rides.

TACTILE MODULATION

- Avoiding putting hands in a bowl to knead or mix ingredients.
- Inability to tolerate a baking mix or splashes of food on hands.
- Limited tolerance for queuing.
- Strong reaction to being bumped or brushed past.
- Under/over dressing for the weather.
- Extreme responses to hot or cold sensations.
- Heightened reactions or minimal reactions to pain.

VISUAL MODULATION

- Blinking or reacting strongly when lights are switched on.
- Preference for keeping curtains closed or wearing sunglasses.
- Closing their eyes to complete tasks to reduce visual input.
- Difficulties tolerating busy environments – this may include high numbers of people moving around, or environments that have significant volumes of visual information in the form of objects or décor.

AUDITORY MODULATION

- A need to wear headphones or ear defenders when going out.
- Avoidance of busy places (note this could also relate to other sensory inputs).
- Strong autonomic reactions to unexpected sounds such as a baby crying or an alarm sounding.
- Requesting the volume of a radio or television be lowered or raised to enable them to tolerate the noise (n.b. this is outside the context of a hearing impairment).

Considerations for goal setting

Developing meaningful goals with your clients is important to agree the aims of your work together, to help identify when your aims have been achieved, and to support measuring of outcomes. There are a range of approaches and resources to support goal setting, with many relating to the principles of SMART goals, that is, goals that are specific, measurable, achievable, relevant and time-bound. Agreeing goals when completing sensory-based intervention is no different in many ways, as your overall goal should remain focused on what will be achieved in terms of functioning or wellbeing as a result of the intervention. After all, if the sensory differences someone is experiencing do not prevent them from doing something or impact on their wellbeing, then the question should be asked, 'Is intervention necessary?' This will require you as a therapist to step back and consider what the underlying sensory or motor components are that are preventing your client from doing what they want to or need to do.

The setting of proximal and distal goals has often been recommended in the sensory integration (SI) literature as a way to capture the connection between these two elements. Within this format your distal goal is the functional change you hope to see, that is, what your client will be able to do if intervention is successful. Your proximal goal should relate to the changes in sensory processing that will help them to achieve that goal. Use of proximal and distal goals helps you to take both a top-down and a bottom-up perspective, that is, one that considers the occupational outcome and the underlying changes. While both of these should be discussed and agreed with your client, making the connection between the proximal and distal factors is likely to call on your professional judgement as the therapist. However, the use of proximal and distal goals can provide a powerful tool to illustrate the rationale for sensory-based interventions and to begin developing your client's, and potentially those who work with them or care for them, understanding of the connection between difficulties they have been experiencing in their occupations and sensory processing.

There are a range of helpful resources available to support goal setting in clinical practice, so rather than discussing this in detail here, a number of tips are provided that should be considered when developing your goals.

- Make sure your goal focuses on what will be achieved, not how they will get there.
    - To be motivating, a goal should help your client envisage the end point or aim of intervention. Goals that instead relate to them

engaging in the intervention should be captured in steps or actions towards that goal.

- Consider all relevant viewpoints.
    - This could include family, carers, service providers and commissioners.
    - While the wishes of your client are paramount, for them to be successful in meeting their aims the support and investment of others, such as family members, carers or support staff, is often also needed.
    - There may also be priorities that have to be considered due to commissioning, such as progressing to a new placement or the remit of the service you can provide.

- Write your goals with your client and in words they would use.
    - This relates primarily to distal goals, which capture the functional aims, but it is important to make sure your client is clear on the relationship between this and your proximal goal, and understand why the changes in sensory processing will help them to achieve their overall goal.
    - Once written, 'sense-check' your goals with your client for unnecessary terminology that lacks personalization, such as referring to 'ADLs' or 'activities of daily living'.

- Consider if it is possible to know when the goal has been achieved.
    - This helps to increase motivation but also allows for outcome measurement, which is likely to be important from both a client and a service perspective.

- Use approach goals rather than avoidance goals.
    - Goals with a positive focus on an achievement rather than a reduction or cessation in a behaviour or problem are naturally more motivating and have been suggested to have a positive impact on wellbeing (Sakaki et al., 2024).
    - While a reduction in a certain difficulty could be an important aim for someone, this can also easily lead to self-blame and guilt when lapses occur.

Table 8.1 Overview of assessment options and criteria for use

Assessment	Format	Age range	Time to administer	Areas considered	Training needed
Adolescent/Adult Sensory Profile (Brown & Dunn, 2002)	Self-report or carer report. Therapist scored	11 years upwards	20–30 minutes	Modulation of taste/smell, touch, visual, auditory and movement input (vestibular and proprioceptive). Also considers impact on activity levels	Training not needed to administer but necessary to accurately interpret
Adult/Adolescent Sensory History (May-Benson, 2015)	Self-report or carer report. Abridged version. Accompanying medical & developmental history form. Includes scoring software	13–95 years old	20–30 minutes	Sensory discrimination, sensory modulation, postural-ocular skills, praxis and social-emotional functioning	Training not needed to administer but necessary to accurately interpret
Sensory Processing Measure, Second Edition (SPM-2) (Parham et al., 2021)	Self-report or carer report. Available to send electronically or paper version. Includes scoring software	21–87 years old (Adolescent form covers 12–21 years old)	15–20 minutes	Modulation and perception of visual, auditory, touch, taste and smell, proprioception, balance and motion (vestibular) input. Also planning and ideas (praxis) and social participation	Training not needed to administer but necessary to accurately interpret

cont.

Assessment	Format	Age range	Time to administer	Areas considered	Training needed
Observations Based on Sensory Integration Theory (Blanche, 2010)	Non-standardized assessment with norms available for comparison	Norms available for ages up to 8 years on certain tests	20–30 minutes	Proprioceptive processing, postural, vestibular functioning and praxis	Post-graduate training in sensory integration required to administer and interpret
Evaluation in Ayres Sensory Integration (EASI) (Mailloux, et al., 2018)	Therapist-administered assessment with standardized and non-standardized sub-tests	3–12 years old	1.5–2 hours	Sensory perception, postural/ocular/bilateral motor integration, praxis and sensory reactivity	Post-graduate training in sensory integration required as well as specific training in administration of this test
Structured Observations of Sensory Integration – Motor (SOSI-M) and Complete Observations of Proprioception (COP-R) (Blanche et al., 2021)	Therapist-administered standardized assessment (outside standardization if used with adults)	5–14 years old	20–40 minutes	Sensory-based motor skills – proprioception, vestibular processing, motor planning and postural control	Requires post-graduate training in sensory integration to administer and interpret

CONCLUSION/KEY LEARNING

This chapter provides an overview of a range of assessments available to support the assessment of sensory integration and alternative ways to assess where no suitable assessment is available. Agreed goals should be designed to support client motivation and focus, as well as helping to capture the success of intervention.

Key points

- Sensory assessment results should be considered in the context of impact on functioning and occupational engagement.
- Assessment in mental health should not be limited to modulation and should consider the full scope of sensory processing difficulties.
- An awareness of potential complicating factors such as medication side effects and symptomology such as hallucinations is needed to support completion and interpretation of assessments.

CHAPTER 9

Levels of Intervention

REBECCA MATSON

When first starting to use interventions that fall within the remit of sensory integration or sensory-based approaches, therapists can often struggle with identifying the level at which they are working, and having confidence in what it may be appropriate to do while working within their scope of practice. This is further complicated by variations and limited consistency in how the terms and descriptors for different approaches are used within the literature. Brown et al. (2018) suggest that one reason for variation in terminology is the evolving nature of understanding and use of concepts such as sensory modulation. However, as they discuss, it is important in supporting evidence-based practice to have a shared understanding. Being able to identify and communicate the terms used to describe different sensory interventions we might use to others is important in providing clarity of expectations and considering potential outcomes as a result of the intervention. This distinction is also an issue that has become important within the literature to improve the integrity of the evidence base to support different sensory intervention approaches.

This chapter forms an introductory overview to the areas of intervention within this book and is followed by further chapters covering particular areas of sensory intervention in more detail. First, this chapter places the focus on helping you to consider what level of intervention is suitable in view of your level of training and skill, your client's needs and presentation, and the nature of sensory difficulties identified. Often more than one approach may be used at one time, and this may be necessary depending on the results of your assessment. For the purposes of this chapter and book, interventions have been separated into sensory strategies, sensory-based interventions and Ayres Sensory Integration (ASI) therapy.

Sensory strategies

Sensory strategies can be described as interventions that are based upon sensory integration theory but would not adhere to the fidelity of the approach (discussed in more detail below in the section 'Ayres Sensory Integration® Therapy'), and may not be actively seeking to change the underlying cause of sensory processing difficulties. These approaches may be used in response to identified sensory needs such as to help regulate responsivity, or could be used due to factors such as a need for improved emotion regulation or managing alertness levels. Sensory strategies can be used in both ways due to the bidirectional relationship between sensory inputs and our arousal levels (illustrated in Figure 9.1), in which each one may impact the other.

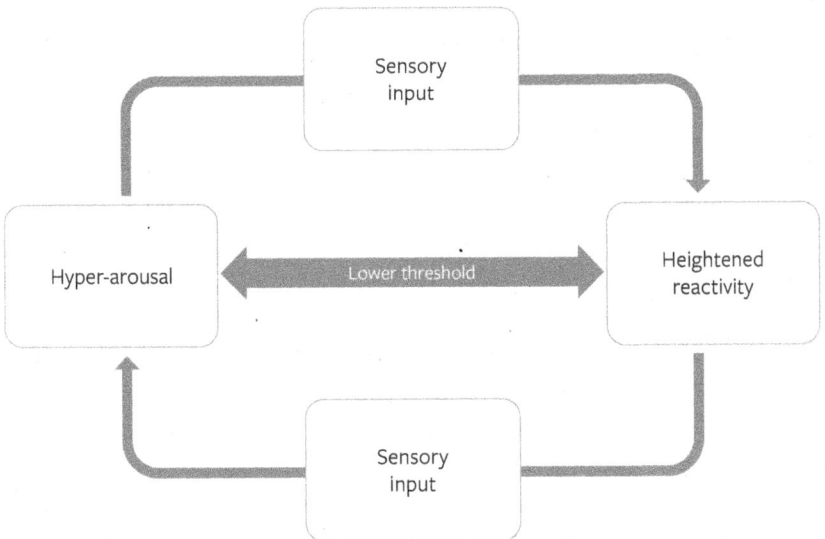

Figure 9.1 Bidirectional relationship between sensory input and arousal levels

Sensory strategies tend to be based upon the principles of sensory modulation, a term used to describe both a process that occurs as part of sensory integration, and an approach that can be taken to intervention. As an intervention, sensory modulation can be described as 'a "bottom up" approach to self-regulation' in which sensory inputs are used to support more adaptive methods of self-management (Hollands et al., 2015, p. 4). These inputs could be provided through equipment, environments or activities. This is an area of intervention from which it could be said everyone may benefit as we all have sensory needs and all naturally use sensory-based strategies of some form at different times, for example having a warm bath to unwind or going for a walk to destress. Using the approach therapeutically is about adding an element of intentionality and supporting someone to identify the sensory inputs they find most regulating and ways to gain these inputs.

Interventions that fall within this remit may be delivered in a direct way, where strategy use is cued by the therapist, or an indirect way, such as suggestions of strategies to trial being agreed with the individual that they can put into practice away from the therapist. This approach can involve varying levels of therapist contact according to client need. A risk with this approach, due to the universality of its applicability, is that clinicians can fall into the trap of a 'one-size-fits-all' approach and provide set items or create a sensory space where there is little scope to adapt according to needs or preferences. We all have different sensory responses and may benefit from different inputs, therefore even when working with someone who does not have any specific sensory processing issues it is important we take the time to consider and respond to their individual patterns. This is where Dunn's (1997) model is particularly helpful. While a formal sensory assessment is not necessarily applicable when using sensory strategies in this way, it is still helpful to use some form of screening tool to help individuals reflect on their own responses and to begin developing ideas for what might be most helpful. A tool such as the Sensory Patterns Questionnaire included in Dunn's *Living Sensationally: Understanding Your Senses* (2009) can be helpful in doing so.

Sensory strategies could be classified as more passive or more active strategies, but overall are much lower demand than more cognitive approaches, making them highly accessible and much easier to use in times of crisis. More passive strategies are those where the person is not required to actively do anything, for example sitting under a weighted blanket, whereas active strategies relate to those that require a response or interaction, such as using a fidget tool, or a movement strategy such as holding a plank position. Both can have a place in an intervention, and in Chapter 10, Sensory Strategies, we will review how to consider which is needed at different times and for different needs.

To support the most effective use of the approach it is important to develop a plan with a person to help consider what strategies may be most effective at what times; and the resource included in Appendix 2 is designed to support you with doing this. Such a plan can be useful both for the person themselves and also for those involved in supporting that person, such as staff or family members, to understand their sensory triggers as well as sensory inputs that are helpful. When in a state of high stress most of us don't immediately think of the strategies that are most helpful to us, and a supporting tool can be beneficial in providing a prompt or reminder, reducing the demands on the person.

Sensory strategies can be used as a more passive approach to sensory stimulation when an individual is less able to engage in developing an individualized plan, but there is a need to provide increased sensory input for a therapeutic purpose or to increase an individual's arousal levels to support engagement. Using this approach does not require any specific sensory processing needs as the intention would be to use increased levels of sensory input to instigate a response rather than responding to an identified under-responsivity. For example, if an individual struggles with fatigue or experiences increased lethargy due to the impact of medication, sensory inputs might be used to help improve focus and alertness. When working on this basis the approach may be much more trial and error and based upon sensations that are commonly thought to be alerting, such as citrus scents or bright lighting. Once identified, strategies may be implemented as part of a routine and could be directed by others, with agreement of the person themselves, such as turning on a bedroom light to help them wake up in the morning. Identifying the strategies that are most helpful for an individual is often an ongoing process that they continue to develop further themselves as they come to better understand the sensations that are most helpful for their own self-regulation.

Environmental adaptations

Considering an individual's environment is always relevant when completing any form of sensory-informed work. We are constantly taking in sensory information from our surroundings without even being consciously aware of it, and this can have a significant impact on our mood and arousal levels. Adaptations to the environment can therefore be an integral part of the intervention process and may support the use of other approaches in practice. This may be particularly relevant when working with individuals residing in an inpatient setting who have very limited control over their environment. Bailliard (2015) describes what he terms 'sensory dissonance', where our environment lacks the sensory cues that would normally support engagement in occupations, leading to heightened levels of distress and disorientation. Part of our intervention may therefore need to include introducing additional sensory cues or compensating for the absence of these in order to facilitate more successful engagement.

An individual's sensory environment will be impacted by both physical and social factors, and intervention may need to incorporate adjustments to both. Common factors that may be considered are detailed in Table 9.1.

Table 9.1 Physical and social environmental factors

Physical adaptations	Social adaptations
Lighting, e.g. dimmer switches, alternative lighting options such as night lights, blackout curtains or blinds	Tone of voice
	Pace of speech
	Use of touch in communication
Reducing or increasing the level of stimulation on walls	Pace of movement – walking not running where possible when responding to an incident
Noise levels – sound proofing, considering location of room if in a shared living environment, alternative alarms that vibrate rather than beep	Avoiding strong scents in perfumes and deodorants
	Using additional verbal cues or prompts to accommodate for the reduction in familiar sensory cues

Depending on an individual's environment, there will be factors that cannot be altered, in which case it may be necessary to consider supports for the person as a way to minimize the impact, such as the use of ear defenders to cope with a noisy environment or a sleep mask to reduce light levels when trying to sleep. Even where there are a number of barriers to altering an individual's environment, the impact of this should always be considered when formulating a plan to support the person and inform understanding of potentially triggering factors. This is discussed further in Chapter 11, Sensory-Informed Approaches.

Sensory-based interventions

A form of intervention that could be described as falling between sensory strategies and higher levels of intervention is sensory-informed protocols that are designed to target particular areas of difficulty and have a standardized administration or protocol, but that would not be considered ASI. An example of this would be the Therapeutic Listening® programme, a sound-based intervention designed to facilitate improved self-organization within the nervous system (Frick & Hacker, 2001), or the Wilbarger approach (Wilbarger & Wilbarger, 1991), which focuses on the treatment of sensory defensiveness. Such approaches require further training and, while they perhaps do not fully align with sensory integration fidelity, utilize sensory properties in order to effect change.

Even if not trained in these approaches yourself, it can be helpful to be aware of when they might be beneficial in order to provide recommendations or to refer on. Such programmes may be indicated to complement other approaches or where ASI is not feasible or not required. Some of the more frequently used protocols will be discussed further in Chapter 11, Sensory-Informed Approaches.

Sensory rooms and spaces

Multi-sensory environments or sensory spaces have been widely utilized with a variety of mental health populations, with suggestions of potential benefits and reasonable efficacy in areas such as regulation of arousal levels and provision of a therapeutic space. Such environments can provide useful spaces for learning sensory strategies and may provide a 'safe space' in a busy ward environment (Doroud et al., 2024; Matson et al., 2021). Sensory rooms have also been suggested to support self-management and replace or reduce the need for restrictive interventions such as physical restraint or additional medication (Doroud et al., 2024). Similar to sensory strategies, a range of people are likely to find them helpful regardless of whether they have any specific sensory processing issues. However, caution is needed in relation to ensuring staff supporting anyone using such a space are provided with suitable training and awareness to avoid assumptions, such as that the same items within the room and the same levels of stimulation will be beneficial to everyone. This will be discussed further in Chapter 11, Sensory-Informed Approaches.

Multi-sensory spaces for individuals with dementia can hold a slightly different focus, where the aim is often for sensory stimulation to support regulation of arousal but also improve cognition. Collier et al. (2010) discuss how providing increased multi-sensory stimulation can support improved functional performance when working with those with dementia by reducing demand on the central nervous system and what she describes as 'cognitive noise'. An important point she does suggest is that in order for this to be effective, it should be informed by an understanding of the individual's sensory needs based on an assessment such as the Adolescent/Adult Sensory Profile (Brown & Dunn, 2002). Further information on the utility of such spaces is provided in Chapter 7, Dementia.

Ayres Sensory Integration® Therapy

Ayres Sensory Integration (ASI) is an approach that adheres to specific fidelity requirements and is tailored in response to needs identified through a comprehensive assessment process. Use of ASI requires formal post-graduate training to a certain level, as identified by one of the sensory integration training providers; the exact level varies according to provider. ASI is based upon principles initially developed by Jean Ayres and would only be used in response to identified sensory processing needs, with the intention being to improve sensory integration and, as a result, areas such as functional performance and self-regulation. Attempts to more firmly distinguish this level of intervention from other sensory interventions have increased in recent years in order to protect and develop the integrity of the evidence base.

The Ayres Sensory Integration Fidelity Measure (ASIFM) (Parham et al., 2011) was developed for this purpose to support both efficacy of intervention and research potential by manualizing the approach and requirements to identify an intervention as ASI. There are a number of challenges to manualizing an intervention that by nature contains high levels of variability according to individual needs, but the measure captures those areas of congruity considered central to the approach. The ASIFM contains both structural elements relating to the environment in which therapy is conducted and therapist qualifications and supports, and process elements which identify components that should be present in an intervention session.

As the fidelity measure was developed in relation to therapy with children in a clinic setting, there are undoubtedly challenges to meeting fidelity when working within adult mental health settings, a number of which will be considered in Chapter 12, Ayres Sensory Integration®. One thing it is important to mention here though is that these barriers do not necessarily prevent adherence to fidelity but require greater creativity on the part of the therapist to adapt and develop ways to achieve it within alternative settings. Therapists working with adults are now using a range of settings and resources in order to meet the different components of fidelity in the aim of meeting their clients' needs.

Summary of levels of intervention

Table 9.2 provides guidance as to when the different levels of intervention could be considered and the level of training required to utilize the intervention. While a number of the interventions do not require a specific level of training, an introductory level of training as well as access to a practitioner who has completed a higher level of training in sensory integration would be beneficial to support the most effective use. Key to all interventions is observation of the responses of your client and an active responsivity to this. We are all sensory beings and will naturally gravitate towards or away from sensory experiences depending on our preferences, so trust these reactions in your client group.

Table 9.2 Different levels of sensory interventions

Intervention level	Sensory-based approaches	Sensory-informed protocols	Environmental adaptations	Sensory stimulation approaches	Ayres Sensory Integration
Examples	Sensory strategies, sensory diet/support plans	Wilbarger approach, Therapeutic Listening	Increase in sensory cues or reduction in sensory stimulation within the environment	Multi-sensory environments (MSEs)	Ayres Sensory Integration therapy measured according to fidelity
When to consider use	Beneficial to all. An individual does not need to have an identified sensory processing difficulty to benefit from using sensory strategies	Protocols are focused on specific identified difficulties with sensory processing and therefore would only be used in response to this	Beneficial to all. We are all impacted by sensory aspects within our environments and the impact will vary depending on our natural preferences	To provide increased or decreased levels of stimulation according to need	Following a comprehensive assessment by a suitably qualified practitioner that has identified a significant sensory processing difficulty
Training required	No specific training required to use these interventions, but use should be informed by awareness of the sensory systems and impact of sensory input on arousal levels. Consider completion of an introductory course in sensory processing prior to commencing use	Formal training in the specific interventions is required to use in practice. Basic training in sensory integration would also be beneficial to support use	No specific training required, but advisory to support suitable adaptations. Consider an introductory course in sensory processing to support application of basic principles and inform appropriate adaptations according to need	No specific training required, but advisory. Sensory equipment companies are able to advise on items to be included to meet specific needs, but will not have detailed knowledge of your specific client group	Specific post-graduate training and ongoing mentoring from a therapist qualified in the approach is a requirement

CONCLUSION/KEY LEARNING

This chapter provides an initial overview of the different levels of sensory-based interventions that are discussed in the following chapters. Being clear on your intervention approach helps you feel confident that it is a fit for your client's needs and within your scope of practice.

Key points

- The approach to intervention should be identified based upon client need and in view of your level of training and competency.
- Interventions should be individualized and there is no one-size-fits-all approach.
- Supervision from a sensory integration practitioner with a higher level of training may aid you in identifying the most suitable approach.

CHAPTER 10

Sensory Strategies

REBECCA MATSON

The use of sensory strategies has grown significantly within mental health settings in recent years, and has become a relatively well accepted part of an individual's crisis plan or de-escalation approach in many places. Sensory strategies are an approach that is relevant to all regardless of the presence of any diagnosis or particular difficulties, as we all use different strategies or activities on a daily basis for the sensory benefits they hold, even if we are not consciously aware of this benefit at the time. As Dunn (2001, p. 618) describes, all of us have our own sensory needs or responses and 'sensory processing patterns are reflections of who we are' rather than any specific pathology or condition. The key is learning how to understand our own responses and consciously utilize those inputs and strategies that are most beneficial to us at different times.

Often the clients we work with in mental health settings already use certain strategies for their sensory benefits, but these can include what could be considered maladaptive strategies, such as self-harm, where that individual is inadvertently seeking a form of sensory input without being fully aware that this is one of the reasons for doing this. For example, punching a wall could be an example of seeking proprioceptive feedback. Therefore, a helpful starting point for using sensory strategies can be identifying the benefits an individual obtains through more harmful strategies and beginning to replace these with strategies that provide the same inputs or benefits but in a way that isn't harmful. It is important to keep in mind, however, that while that person may have obtained specific sensory inputs through such strategies, the sensory input does not necessarily need to be an exact match. The ultimate benefit of any sensory input tends to be the effect it has within the brain in supporting regulation, and for any one person there may be various sensory inputs that facilitate this effect. Therefore, it is important to complete a broader screening of sensory needs and responses when considering and identifying alternative strategies.

Sensory strategies have been incorporated within a number of initiatives or guidance documents in relation to mental health settings in acknowledgement of their benefits, from supporting self-management to reducing the use of more restrictive interventions, with this influence being apparent in Australia (Australian Health Ministers' Advisory Council, 2013; Wright et al., 2022), New Zealand (Azuela et al., 2023), America and the UK (Haig & Hallett, 2023; Scanlan & Novak, 2015). Such approaches have been advocated by various initiatives, such as being part of 'calm down methods' in Safe Wards (Safe Wards, 2023). A significant benefit of such approaches has been noted to be the collaborative and client-led focus that has the potential to make such strategies more sustainable in the long term, and transferable from an inpatient setting to the community (Keptner et al., 2021; Matson et al., 2021; Wallis et al., 2018).

The aim of this chapter is to help you consider the ways in which sensory strategies may be of use within your practice and how to begin identifying which strategies to consider and when.

The evidence for using sensory strategies in mental health

The vast majority of research within mental health has been focused on this level of sensory intervention rather than higher-level approaches such as more formalized Ayres Sensory Integration. This has included consideration of sensory rooms or spaces, as well as sensory boxes or kits, and specific items of equipment such as weighted blankets (Craswell et al., 2021; Haig & Hallett, 2023; Matson et al., 2021; Scanlan & Novak, 2015). While currently there continues to be a need for more conclusive evidence in relation to the effectiveness of such approaches, some of the main benefits identified within the literature include increased self-management, supporting empowerment and reducing the need for more restrictive interventions (Alhaj & Trist, 2023; Craswell et al., 2021; Lindberg et al., 2019).

Certain factors have been suggested to increase the effectiveness of the approach, such as education of the person themselves and those supporting them on a day-to-day basis to use the strategies (Craswell et al., 2021; Scanlan & Novak, 2015). Other important factors include personalization of strategies based on individual need, and accessibility of the strategies as and when needed (Craswell et al., 2021; Matson et al., 2021). Therefore, it may be important to ensure that where possible use of strategies does not depend solely on access to a certain space such as a sensory room and that ongoing use of the strategies is affordable for that person.

Sensory diets or plans

'Sensory diet' is a term used to describe a plan to structure or integrate the use of different sensory inputs into a daily routine or programme at set intervals that is personalized to each individual based upon their sensory needs (Champagne & Pfeiffer, 2020; Wilbarger & Wilbarger, 2020). This can include the use of different items or particular activities or environments in order to support overall regulation and can be either directed by the person themselves or by supporting staff. It is often supported with a sensory kit or sensory box containing items to facilitate implementation of agreed strategies or activities. Champagne and Pfeiffer (2020) describe that one of the benefits of this within mental health is that it supports an increased level of control over the sensory inputs the person experiences within their day-to-day routine and occupations.

Sensory diets have been used within mental health to support regulation of sensory defensiveness (Moore & Henry, 2002), trauma/PTSD (Champagne, 2011; Kimball, 2023; Kimball et al., 2018) and anxiety (Pfeiffer & Kinnealey, 2003). While the term can have unhelpful connotations, such as the suggestion of a prescribed nature, the ideas or strategies that would be incorporated into a sensory diet can also be added into a broader sensory plan or a safety tool to create a more integrated approach with other forms of strategies. While the name used may vary, having a format to guide strategy use tends to be highly useful within mental health, particularly to support maintenance of a desirable arousal state and move away from solely using strategies in a reactive way. For example, periods of physical activity to support overall regulation could be scheduled, or use of a regulating strategy could be encouraged before a time of day that tends to be difficult for that person.

Within this book the broader term 'sensory plan' is used to capture this area while allowing for more flexibility in the exact format of this. A template to support development of a sensory plan is provided within the appendices, but this is likely to benefit from further adaptation depending upon setting and client group. It is important to remember that sensory needs can change and therefore a sensory plan should be reviewed on a regular basis to ensure it remains appropriate to need. It is advisable to set an identified review period, such as six months, but to review sooner should there be notable changes such as alterations in risk profile or a significant improvement or decline in mental health.

Considering the benefits of the different senses
Vestibular strategies

When considering vestibular strategies, it is important to remember the different forms of vestibular input and the differing impacts they may have on someone. Vestibular input can be highly effective in calming or alerting, but caution is also needed as there can be a small difference between the amount that is helpful for someone and that is enough to alter their arousal levels beyond what is desired (Lane et al., 2019). In general, linear vestibular input provided at a steady pace is calming for the majority of people, and rotational or variable vestibular input is alerting. However, ensure you consider individual sensory processing patterns and sensitivities carefully and alter the level of challenge accordingly. For example, if someone has a strong vestibular sensitivity it does not mean the input can't be therapeutic for them, but that it would need to be provided in a certain way, such as a well-supported and controlled rocking chair rather than sitting and bouncing on a gym ball with no back. Identifying ways to gain higher levels of vestibular input is more of a challenge for adults, but below are some ideas of ways in which it can be incorporated into sensory plans.

LINEAR VESTIBULAR INPUT

- Using a rocking chair or gaming chair can provide an alternative.
- Sitting and bouncing on a gym ball.
- Running.
- Swimming provides vestibular input in combination with other regulating sensations such as proprioception, which helps to regulate response.
- Yoga poses that involve inverting the head.
- Going for a drive.
- Using a hammock or swing.

ROTATIONAL VESTIBULAR INPUT

- Dancing where there are moves that require spinning.
- Activities such as go-karting.
- Fairground rides such as waltzers (a ride containing separate cars that rotate on a turntable).
- Spinning on a desk chair.

Proprioceptive strategies

Proprioception has the most immediate effect on our brain stem and therefore is highly powerful in regulation and supports the processing of other senses (Blanche & Schaaf, 2001). Therefore, while items that help to provide proprioception often can't fit in a sensory box or kit, it is important to incorporate strategies into a sensory plan that use this sense. Where no items are needed, or where the items are too large to be kept in a kit, prompt cards can be used to remind the individual to consider using the strategies at different times. Proprioception can be provided in a range of ways and does not need to depend on available equipment; for example, one of the most effective ways can be through body-weight exercises. Proprioception can be gained through any strategies that require heavy muscle work, so the possibilities of ways in which this can be achieved are endless. Below are some examples:

- Holding a plank. The intensity can also be increased through varying the approach to lift alternating hands.
- Doing press-ups, wall push-ups or chair press-ups.
- Yoga poses with high levels of stretch. Consider adding cards with instructions or diagrams to a sensory kit.
- Weights-based exercises, for example using dumbbells, kettlebells or powerbags, depending on risk assessment and level of muscle tension desired.
- Progressive muscle relaxation using either a script or an app.
- Gardening tasks such as digging.
- Household tasks such as vacuuming.
- Pushing a gym ball against a wall or against another person – this allows variation of the amount of muscle tension used.
- Chewing chewing gum or chewy sweets.
- Squeezing a hand exerciser or firm stress ball can be used to provide intense muscle tension in the arms.
- Squeezing Theraputty.
- Using a treadmill on a higher gradient.
- Using a cross trainer on higher resistance.
- Stretching with a Theraband.

Taste and olfactory strategies

Our sense of taste and smell are closely connected, which is why these two senses are discussed together here and tend to be clustered within sensory assessments such as the ASH (May-Benson, 2015). Our sense of smell has a direct connection to our emotions and memories, which can make it both highly triggering and also highly effective in quickly grounding and calming (Kontaris et al., 2020). Use of strategies in relation to particular aromas or scents can therefore be powerful and are worth considering for anyone you are working with in developing a sensory plan or kit. Due to the potentially triggering nature of scents, caution is advised when initially trialling these, particularly if working with someone with a known history of trauma, but as with any strategy, allowing that person to guide and feel in control of the process is a good strategy for minimizing this risk.

TASTE STRATEGIES

Stronger tastes tend to be more effective for grounding or increasing alertness and more subtle flavours for calming.

- Extra-strong mints or peppermints.
- Sour sweets.
- Biting into a lemon.
- Spicy foods.
- Milky drinks.
- Fizzy drinks.

OLFACTORY STRATEGIES

- Aromatherapy oils in different scents. Response can vary according to preference, but citrus and mint scents tend to be more alerting and floral scents such as lavender more calming.
- Creating a water-based spray with a preferred scent helps to make aromatherapy oils a more portable strategy.
- Scented shower gels or bath foam.
- Hand creams in a calming scent.
- Using a laundry detergent in a preferred scent.
- Scented wheat bags or cushions.
- Room sprays or diffusers.
- Candles.

Tactile strategies

The sense of touch is fundamental to our wellbeing due to strong connections with attachment and regulation (Ayres, 2005; Duhn, 2010). When considering touch strategies, it is important to keep in mind the different forms of touch, particularly light touch experiences, which tend to be more alerting or triggering, and deep pressure touch, which for most people is more regulating or calming. Both can have their uses, as if you are working with someone who is low in arousal and attempting to develop strategies to support an increase in this, light touch strategies are likely be more effective, whereas if the primary need is to support greater regulation of arousal and reducing the overall arousal state then deep pressure touch is much more likely to have the desired effect. However, some caution may be needed when using deep pressure touch strategies with individuals who have experienced trauma as deep pressure can have an apparently incongruent effect to that which may be expected due to previous traumatic experiences and can be dysregulating for certain individuals (Koomar, 2009).

There are a number of ways in which touch experiences can be used effectively in practice to support regulation, and while more expensive items such as a weighted blanket are perhaps the most well-known way of providing deep pressure touch, there are various lower-cost options that can have a positive effect. Below are different strategy ideas for using light touch and deep pressure touch that may be useful within mental health settings.

DEEP PRESSURE TOUCH

- Weighted shawl or blanket. A shawl may be beneficial when there is a need for the strategy to be portable or of lower intensity.
- Using massage tools – a particular benefit is that an individual can alter the amount of pressure applied.
- Hand massage – either self-administered or by someone else.
- Wearing Lycra sports clothing provides more constant tactile input.
- Wearing fitted clothing such as slim jeans.
- A filled hot water bottle can help provide a weighted sensation.
- Microwavable animals are often filled with pellets that give a gentle weighted sensation.
- Using a vibration cushion. While vibration is not deep pressure it activates the same tactile pathway and therefore can be a helpful alternative to trial.

LIGHT TOUCH

- Using a koosh ball.
- Rolling water beads around the hand or putting the hand into a tub of them.

- Plunging the hand into tubs of rice or lentils or allowing them to run over the fingers.

Visual strategies

Visual input can be particularly problematic when an individual resides in an environment over which they have minimal control, or when attempting to access new places where visual stimuli can easily become overwhelming. Consider the different environments individuals may access and the impact of factors such as different lighting, bright colours or busy walls on arousal level. Also consider how most people naturally arrange their environment to include preferred visual input such as to be very colourful or very plain, or how a certain scene can be immediately calming for someone. Therefore, when considering visual strategies, this may entail helping an individual to alter the level of visual stimulation within their own environment, or to manage their response to visual input they encounter in other environments. Potential visual strategies to consider when developing a sensory plan include:

- the ability to vary levels of lighting, for example by using a dimmer switch, according to the desired level of arousal
- night lights or star projectors – these are often useful when individuals find complete darkness difficult to tolerate
- fibre optics
- wearing sunglasses to reduce glare from natural or artificial light
- adding pictures of calming scenes to a sensory box or kit
- identifying places that are visually calming and adding suggestions to visit them to a sensory plan
- dressing in clothing in preferred colours, or colours that help the person feel more alert or calmer.

Auditory strategies

Similar to visual input, noise can be problematic for individuals with mental health conditions for a number of reasons, and management of this is often an important consideration when attempting to increase interaction; for accessing different places or locations; and supporting overall wellbeing. Therefore, strategies to manage the level or type of auditory input within an individual's environment are often part of a sensory kit or plan. Another way in which auditory strategies can be important is in the use of music to facilitate changes in arousal or mood. Many people use music to alter their mood or facilitate engagement in different activities; for example, faster-paced music or music with a strong beat is often used in a setting such as an exercise class to help people to feel more energized.

There are a few common approaches to support management of the level of noise when this is not within that individual's control:

- ear defenders or ear plugs
- white noise – this can be provided through a white noise machine or an app on a phone
- playing preferred music on headphones to block out other problematic noise.

When using music as a strategy, while certain aspects tend to have a similar effect on the majority of people, it is important to remember that response can also be quite individualized and to take time getting to know each individual's personal preferences and responses. While classical music may be calming for one person, for another who does not enjoy it there could be a different effect. Music or particular songs can bring back memories and remind us of a particular experience or time, therefore we need to keep in mind the very personal connection it can have.

When adding music to a sensory plan or box it is therefore important to consider identifying songs or types of music that help to evoke different emotions or responses and can be used to alter mood in a helpful way. When adding this to a plan try to identify music according to different emotions such as being sad, angry, happy or lethargic, or according to different activities that person needs to be able to do and what helps them alter their arousal state in order to do so. Music can be used in a cathartic way but can also be used to indulge an unhelpful mood, so a starting point may need to be developing an understanding of how each person uses different types of music.

Considerations for developing a sensory kit

As sensory kits or plans may be used with anyone, not just those with identified sensory processing difficulties, the same level of assessment is not necessarily needed as for other sensory approaches, but it is still helpful as a starting point to develop an understanding of each person's sensory preferences and responses. This may be done through use of a checklist that identifies a range of potential strategies in relation to the different senses or could be done through gradual trialling of a variety of items in relation to each sense. A mixture of both approaches is likely to be the most helpful approach in order to develop a kit that best suits a person's individual needs.

A sensory kit is best accompanied by a plan that helps either the individual themselves identify when different strategies are likely to be most helpful, or helps others involved in supporting them to direct them to use strategies. While each individual may have particularly positive responses to certain sensory experiences, it is most helpful to identify strategies in relation to all of the senses to provide a range of potential options and inputs depending on the particular need at the time. Depending on an individual's particular needs, their plan may well include a higher number of movement-based strategies, for example, but they are likely to also benefit from other accessible strategies to alter their arousal when not able to use movement strategies.

When first developing a sensory plan or kit it is advisable to monitor responses either through the person themselves keeping a log and reviewing what has been helpful at what times, or through you as the therapist supporting them in initially trialling each strategy so you can observe the response and impact on their arousal. How this is approached is likely to depend on a range of factors, such as whether it is an inpatient service or community team and the level of understanding that person has of their sensory patterns and arousal levels. A sensory plan or kit is unlikely to stay the same as when it is first set up and will evolve as that person continues to use the strategies; certain ones may change in effectiveness or, based upon those that work for them, they may identify further strategies that provide similar inputs. One of the most rewarding benefits of developing a sensory kit is seeing the gradual development in self-understanding as the person begins to add new strategies and gains a deeper awareness of their own needs.

Perhaps the most important point to remember is that everyone is an individual and will have individual sensory patterns and responses. While certain sensory strategies are commonly thought to be calming and others alerting, this is not always the case and varies from person to person, which is why the strategies within this chapter have not been separated into calming and alerting. Guidance is provided above on caution that may be needed in relation to different types of sensory input and potential effects, but it is important to trial strategies with your clients and evaluate individual responses and preferences to develop a plan that is likely to be most effective for them. A sensory kit or box should never be given to someone without consideration of their individualized responses and there is no 'one-size-fits-all' ready-to-issue sensory kit.

Another factor to consider is risk assessment in relation to different strategies and items that may be used within the sensory kit. This will require careful consideration on the part of the therapist to balance management of risk with risk enablement where a strategy or activity is likely to have therapeutic benefits. While depending on the setting there may be certain environmental or procedural restrictions on what can be provided or used, outside of this always try to balance the potential value of the strategy with the potential risks of the item. When considering this a helpful process to follow is the Royal College of Occupational Therapists (2018) risk enablement process contained within their *Embracing Risk; Enabling Choice* guidance to help you ensure you have fully considered risk but also the potential benefits. While the process focuses on risk-assessing activities, it is easily transferable to assessing use of a sensory item and also helps you consider all the necessary stages, starting with identifying the value of the strategy, and then considering and assessing the risks, developing plans for enablement and completing regular reviews.

Risk considerations

While it is beyond the scope of this chapter to provide an extensive list of the risks of all possible items, Table 10.1 outlines the risks of items commonly used with adults in mental health settings to help start the risk enablement process. A helpful starting point when assessing the risk of items you are considering issuing is the manufacturer instructions or guidelines, as the risk of items can depend on the nature of the materials and factors such as whether they are non-toxic.

Table 10.1 Potential risks of commonly used sensory items

Strategy or item	Risks	Potential adjustments
Weighted blanket or shawl	Overheating, skin integrity, medication side effects that increase lethargy, low muscle tone, fire safety, infection control	Ensure weight is no more than 10% of body weight – where this is exceeded the rationale for this requires careful consideration and clear documentation Supervise initial use to ensure the person can remove the blanket for themselves Consider purchasing items with higher fire safety for inpatient environments Where a blanket may be used by multiple people a wipeable blanket or blanket with changeable covers is recommended for infection control RCOT (2023) recommend a personalized risk assessment that identifies guidance such as time period for use of the blanket, individual responses that may suggest the blanket should be removed, and level of support required where relevant

cont.

Strategy or item	Risks	Potential adjustments
Gym ball	Falls, bursting, over/under-inflation, wear and tear, exceeding weight allowance	Complete a visual check for punctures prior to each use Identify the required size with the person – this should support 90° flexion at the knee Recommend anti-burst balls Where an individual has weaker core stability or balance, consider using a peanut ball as an alternative Check the need for inflation prior to each use
Theraputty	Ingestion/choking, skin irritation, over-exertion	Check manufacturer guidance to ensure it is non-toxic Consider supervised use if ingestion is a potential risk Most Theraputty is non-toxic and latex free so skin irritation is unlikely, but as a precaution, checking known allergies is advisable
Aromatherapy oils	Allergic reaction, contraindication for medications, strong emotional reaction, ingestion	Caution when using oils on a diffuser in shared environments as it could have a different impact for different people Consult with a doctor or pharmacist about potential contraindications with different medications Avoid contact with eyes Avoid steam inhalation where an individual has asthma
Theraband	Breakage during use, ligature, over-exertion	Complete a visual check of condition prior to use Identify the most suitable resistance level for that person Supervised use only if a ligature risk; or use may be prohibited fully where this is the case Consult GP/doctor if the individual is minimally physically active
Weights	Over-exertion, muscle strain	Consider consulting a personal trainer/gym instructor to support development of an exercise plan Review by GP may be needed if this is a new activity for that person or if they have previously been physically inactive
Tangle fidgets and other small fidget items	Ingestion, inserting of items, breakage	Check manufacturer guidance to ensure the product is non-toxic Supervised use only may be considered where there is a higher risk Inspect the items for small pieces or potential issues such as sharp plastic prior to issuing

CONCLUSION/KEY LEARNING

Sensory strategies have been suggested to support increased self-management and empowerment of clients, as well as helping to reduce the use of restrictive practices. This chapter provides an overview of the purpose and potential utility of sensory strategies, as well as a range of ideas for implementation in practice.

Key points

- Identification of sensory strategies should be guided by each individual and their responses and preferences.
- Transferability and accessibility of strategies is key in supporting ongoing use and effectiveness.
- Risk enablement, and considering both the potential risks and benefits of a strategy, is an important part of the process.

CHAPTER 11

Sensory-Informed Approaches

REBECCA MATSON

There are a number of approaches used in practice that require a certain level of knowledge and application of principles of sensory integration, but without being described as sensory integration therapy. Within this chapter various interventions will be considered that are perhaps more prescribed or therapist-led in nature, some of which require additional specific training to use in practice. It is important that therapists are clear on the nature of the interventions that they use in practice to ensure they are working within our scope of practice but also to protect the integrity of different interventions and their evidence base. While the interventions discussed within this chapter all relate to sensory integration theory, they would not be considered Ayres Sensory Integration and it is important to be clear on that point.

The aim within this chapter is to provide you with sufficient information to consider the relevance of different sensory-informed approaches to your client group and where it may be worthwhile considering additional training to utilize these. Not all of the approaches discussed within this chapter require additional specific training but there are important considerations in the use of each which will be discussed within this chapter. The current state of evidence for the different approaches in relation to mental health will also be considered.

Wilbarger approach (Wilbarger & Wilbarger, 1991)

The Wilbarger approach, sometimes known as the Wilbarger Protocol or the Wilbarger brushing programme, is focused on intervention for sensory defensiveness. While the approach is thought to have specific benefits for tactile defensiveness, it is not used exclusively for this area of difficulty and is thought to have broader potential to support self-regulation (Wilbarger & Wilbarger, 2020). This is due to the use of deep pressure touch and proprioceptive input in the techniques, which are two of the 'power senses' in sensory integration that have been identified as having specific benefits for supporting overall regulation and organization. The approach contains three main components as outlined by Wilbarger and Wilbarger (2020):

- Education in relation to sensory defensiveness and its impact. This could be to the person themselves or those supporting them in administration of the programme.
- A sensory diet or plan which integrates prescribed activities at certain intervals throughout the day. This component is not discussed in detail here as it is a component often used outside of the Wilbarger approach and is therefore covered within Chapter 10, Sensory Strategies.
- A therapist-administered intervention programme, usually in the form of brushing and joint compression.

Utilization of this approach requires specific training to ensure the different components are administered in a certain way, particularly the brushing and joint compression. The therapist-administered component involves the use of a specific type of brush to apply deep pressure to an individual's arms, back, legs and feet. This is integrated with periods of joint compression to provide proprioceptive input. The intervention is delivered at set intervals throughout the day with ideal time periods between administration being identified as between 90 minutes and two hours (Wilbarger & Wilbarger, 2020). The components of the approach have been developed based upon knowledge of the central nervous system and regulating inputs, so adherence to the recommended components and timings is advocated, which is why specialist training as well as ongoing mentoring in the approach is needed. Wilbarger and Wilbarger (2020) also advise that those using the approach should also have completed training in sensory integration theory to help understand the underlying principles.

While much of the discussion in relation to the approach is focused on children, it has been used with mental health populations and to reduce the impact of anxiety (Kimball et al., 2018; Moore & Henry, 2002; Pfeiffer & Kinnealey, 2003). The approach has been suggested to have potential benefits in regulating sensory defensiveness and related emotion dysregulation, but overall, this is based on small-scale studies and there is a need for greater development of the evidence base for the use of this approach within adult mental health. There is some suggestion that the approach may be effective for women with

PTSD, but studies evaluating this noted variations in response depending on the type of trauma and related symptomology experienced (Kimball et al., 2018). Pfeiffer and Kinnealey's (2003) study focused on adults who experienced sensory defensiveness and connected anxiety but with no psychiatric diagnoses, therefore the results may need to be applied cautiously to a psychiatric population with various comorbidities. The study did show promising results, however, for the potential of the approach in regulating sensory defensiveness and thereby lowering anxiety levels. Due to quite a small and limited evidence base with mental health populations, the approach should be used cautiously, with careful monitoring for any contraindications or adverse reactions.

Therapeutic Listening® (Frick & Hacker, 2001)

The Therapeutic Listening programme is a sensory-based intervention that uses modified music in order to effect changes in sensory processing both specific to the auditory system and broader sensory modulation, as well as bilateral coordination (Frick, 2020). Although the programme primarily utilizes auditory input, its significant impact is thought to occur through the vestibular system due to the close connection between the auditory and vestibular system (Frick, 2020). The vestibular system is central to organizing responses to sensory input, which may explain the programme's potential effectiveness (Ayres, 2005; Lane, 2020b).

There has been suggestion of use of Therapeutic Listening within mental health, but while available studies appear to have adhered to certain principles of the intervention, it is unclear if they followed a specific protocol (Gaur et al., 2021). Balaji et al. (2021) published a protocol for a randomized controlled trial (RCT) considering the use of Therapeutic Listening with adolescents with depression residing in inpatient settings that requires the use of Frick and Hacker's (2021) specific programme, and completion of the required formal training, to administer. However, the results of this RCT do not yet appear to be available, and therefore knowledge regarding the effectiveness of this approach in mental health remains limited. There are also specific contraindications, with Frick (2020) stating that Therapeutic Listening should not be used with those with schizophrenia.

Similar to the Wilbarger approach, Therapeutic Listening requires specialist training to ensure the intervention is delivered in line with established principles and directions, with a central part of the intervention involving listening to the tailored music twice a day, and the length of intervention varying depending on the individual. In order to use the intervention, therapists are required to attend a specific training course and advised to access ongoing mentoring in the approach.

Sensory/Snoezelen™ rooms

The terms 'sensory room' and 'Snoezelen™ room' are often used interchangeably with the difference between the two not always fully clear. A Snoezelen room is a specific type of sensory room that originated in the Netherlands and can perhaps be described as a more controlled multi-sensory environment that is often used with adults who are less able to self-direct the intervention due to the level of cognitive impairment, such as may be the case in more advanced dementia. The intention of these rooms is to aid regulation of arousal or provide increased stimulation in order to support engagement (Collier et al., 2010). 'Sensory room' is a broader term, with the room often having no particular specification but being intended to support the use of sensory-based strategies. Within mental health, sensory rooms have often been used to support de-escalation and prompt the use of identified sensory-based coping strategies (Lindberg et al., 2019; Sutton et al., 2013).

While overall the evidence is inconclusive, a range of studies of the use of sensory rooms within mental health show positive potential benefits for reducing agitation, facilitating engagement with others, and supporting self-regulation (Chalmers et al., 2012; Dorn et al., 2020; Lindberg et al., 2019; Sutton et al., 2013; Wiglesworth & Farnworth, 2016). Sensory rooms have often been advocated as a way to reduce the need for restrictive interventions, and the potential to achieve this has led to increased use in mental health settings (Haig & Hallett, 2023). However, a systematic review by Haig and Hallett (2023) found that evidence to date of a direct connection between sensory room use and a reduction in restrictive interventions such as physical restraint and seclusion is inconclusive. Their review did support previously identified benefits such as emotion regulation and self-management, which are likely to decrease incidents of aggression and self-harm that may lead to the use of restrictive interventions.

There is no set prescription for what such a room should contain, but to maximize potential benefits it is important that they contain a range of sensory strategies to allow the user to personalize the space according to their own individual sensory preferences. Sensory rooms often contain items such as a rocking chair, weighted blanket or shawl, aromatherapy diffuser, projector or variable forms of lighting, small fidget items, bean bags and sometimes items such as colouring books and sour sweets or strong mints. Items in the room tend to be used in a self-directed manner, and one way in which someone can be supported in using the room where needed is to develop a directed plan outlining which items they find beneficial to enable staff support in personalizing the room when the person is in a higher state of arousal and perhaps less able to initiate this themselves.

Due to the potential for personalization, sensory rooms are an intervention that could have applicability for any client. While no specific training is required to support use of a sensory room, undertaking at least introductory training will greatly inform ability to do so and prevent errors that can be commonly made such as directing each person towards the same strategies simply because they have been witnessed to work for someone else. Training also helps to reduce the risk of adverse reactions and can help provide knowledge of how to support someone should they experience an adverse response to a particular sensory item. The importance of staff training has therefore been advocated in a number of studies (Chalmers et al., 2012; Craswell et al., 2021; Scanlan & Novak, 2015).

Principles to consider when developing a sensory room:

- Are items included that provide a range of sensory inputs?
- Is there the ability to personalize the room and alter factors such as the level of lighting, the music playing or silence if preferred, or the choice of seating?
- If in a ward environment, is the room away from the main thoroughfare to reduce the impact of external noises and lighting?
- Risk assessment of the room in view of specific risks within your setting.
- Sustainability of the items included for ongoing use.
- How can clients best be involved in the design, naming and ongoing development of the room?
- How will room use be monitored and reviewed to ensure items are cleaned or replaced as and when necessary?
- Infection control in relation to the items included in view of your specific settings guidance.
- How can the strategies supported by the available items be transferred outside of the room to allow use when accessing other areas, or when no longer able to access the sensory room?

While sensory rooms can be a helpful starting point in enabling an individual to become more aware of their sensory preferences and strategies that are helpful, if consideration is not given to strategies beyond this it can be problematic when an individual is unable to access the room due to someone else using it or when they are discharged from the hospital environment (Matson et al., 2021).

Tina Champagne has provided practical resources to support a number of these considerations on her website OT-Innovations, including an adaptable policy and procedure for use as well as recommended items to include.[1]

Interoception programmes

Interoception relates to our ability to identify and make sense of internal sensations within the body. With interoception gaining increased focus within mental health there is a need for interventions to support addressing this area of concern. Interoceptive difficulties have been identified as a common area of difficulty in a number of mental health conditions, including eating disorders, depression, PTSD and anxiety disorders (Khalsa et al., 2018). Previous focus has generally been on interoceptive programmes for children and is much more widely acknowledged as a common area of difficulty in autism.

One such programme, the Interoception Curriculum (Mahler, 2019), has gained increasing popularity within a range of settings. The programme is designed with children in mind, so the resources are more suited to a younger client group, but it may be possible to adapt it for working with adult populations. It includes a series of lessons focused on developing self-regulation through increasing awareness of body signals and identifying responses to them. The curriculum is available to purchase without the requirement for any specific training, but training may be advisable to implement it successfully. Improving your own understanding of this hidden eighth sense is likely to significantly improve your chance of effectively working on this area with your clients.

Sensory attachment intervention

Sensory attachment intervention (SAI) is an approach developed by Éadaoin Bhreathnach for the treatment of children and adults who have experienced early traumatic experiences including abuse and neglect (Sensory Attachment Intervention, no date). SAI draws on the theory of sensory integration alongside the dynamic maturational model (Crittenden & Landini, 2011) to consider both attachment experiences and alterations in sensory processing. Therapy focuses on the alterations in sensory processing that are thought to result from arousal difficulties and a continuous state of fear caused by these early experiences, but with ongoing evaluation of attachment responses to inform this (Bhreathnach, 2009). Bhreathnach (2018) asserts that if either of these aspects are not

---

1 www.ot-innovations.com

considered in the intervention process then the intervention could become inadvertently triggering due to misinterpretation. Due to this focus intervention sessions would usually involve the primary carer to support coregulation as part of the process.

Currently there is limited published evidence on the use of this approach, with the main sources available being in the form of conference papers or presentations rather than more formalized research or evaluations (Bhreathnach, 2008, 2009, 2018). The intervention, however, is based upon well-established theories as identified above and is likely to greatly support the understanding of therapists working with those who have experienced trauma. SAI requires specialized training in the approach, but with previous training in both sensory integration and the dynamic maturational model being a pre-requisite to complete the training due to the need for this foundational knowledge.

Environmental adaptations

Another area of intervention that may be considered within sensory-informed approaches is the alterations therapists can make, or support an individual to make, to their environment. This may include adaptations to the person's own living environment, such as installing different lighting to regulate visual sensitivity. It could also involve consulting with other relevant parties to facilitate adaptations to other environments a client may access, such as a college or the hospital where they reside. While there are often limitations on what can be done in an environment that is a shared or public space, it is important to consider this as a possibility and advocate for our servicer users wherever possible in this respect. Making such adaptations does not require any further training on the part of the therapist, but a knowledge of the evidence base for the impact of sensory aspects of different environments is likely to support the ability to advocate effectively.

The sensory cues within different environments can be problematic for an individual with a mental health condition but can also be important in facilitating or cuing the ability to engage in a valued occupation (Bailliard, 2015; Bailliard et al., 2023). Bailliard et al. (2023) describe the danger of assuming sensory inputs will have the same impact on a person regardless of the specific environment, and highlight the need to consider how this may vary in order to gain an accurate idea of needs. Adjustments that need to be made in one setting may not be universal, and a therapist will need to consider performance in the different environments for an individual and advise accordingly. This is where an occupational therapist's skill in activity analysis will also be central to the intervention process.

CONCLUSION/KEY LEARNING

This chapter considers a range of interventions that while informed by sensory integration theory to varying extents would not be considered Ayres Sensory Integration. A number of these approaches require specific training: where this is the case it is identified within this chapter.

Key points

- Ensuring you are clear on the applicability and remit of the approach being used is important in supporting evidence-based practice.
- When utilizing multi-sensory environments or sensory rooms, facilitating personalization of the space according to need will help maximize the benefits.
- Adaptations to the sensory qualities of an environment can facilitate positive engagement.

CHAPTER 12

Ayres Sensory Integration®

REBECCA MATSON

Ayres Sensory Integration (ASI) therapy involves the therapeutic use of sensory-motor activities focused on individual need, with the intention of eliciting an adaptive response to environmental demands and thereby enabling skill development (Schaaf & Mailloux, 2015). The approach is dependent on development of a strong therapeutic relationship and provision of the 'just right challenge'; that is, activities that both consider current capabilities and facilitate skill development for a client. Therapy aims to improve the underlying sensory-motor deficits that are impacting on an individual's functioning and participation (Schoen et al., 2019). Using this approach in practice requires the completion of post-graduate training accompanied by engagement in focused mentoring from a qualified ASI practitioner.

ASI has come to be known by this trademarked term in recent years due to a need to distinguish this targeted and focused intervention approach and protect the integrity of the intervention. While formal sensory integration therapy sessions have been used in practice since Jean Ayres first began developing the approach in the 1970s (Watling & Hauer, 2015), there was a lack of clear standards to help identify when this level of therapy was being implemented. Fidelity criteria were needed to support further research into the effectiveness of this level of intervention, but also to provide guidance to clinicians in delivering the intervention in the way intended and that is likely to have the greatest effectiveness. Since the introduction of the Ayres Sensory Integration Fidelity Measure (ASIFM) (Parham et al., 2011), therapists have had specific guidance to consider and implement supported by a checklist to enable reflection on their intervention sessions and consider congruence to ASI principles.

ASI has most frequently been used with child populations, and this is perhaps why some of the principles of intervention, and equipment traditionally used, appear quite childlike. ASI clinic spaces often reflect the roots of the approach with child populations and tend to be brightly coloured, containing a range of equipment such as ball pools and swings, designed to engage the interest and motivation of a child. Careful consideration is needed as to how these spaces may need to be altered when working with adult populations, or whether the use of more varied spaces may be most appropriate to meet the needs of an adult. Later in this chapter we will consider some of the different spaces that may provide the necessary affordances and sensory opportunities but that may be more natural and accessible environments for an adult.

The principles of ASI closely relate to developmental approaches with the aim to alter underlying neurophysiology (Watling & Hauer, 2015), and therefore use could be considered most effective when an individual is in that early intervention period, particularly while the sensory systems are still developing. Having said this, neuroplasticity does not stop when we reach adulthood, and while it is likely that more prolonged intervention may be required to achieve changes in the underlying sensory processing, it is possible, and the brain's response to sensory input can alter and become more adaptive (Cozolino, 2017).

Despite the added complexities, use of ASI is increasing with adult populations, including within adult mental health, in response to a growing awareness of the sensory needs and difficulties of these populations. When looking at the requirements and principles of the approach it can be tempting to rule out this level of intervention due to it being too childlike or time intensive, or requiring equipment that is simply not available within the majority of adult mental health settings, all of which are very real considerations and potential barriers. The aim of this chapter is therefore to help you reflect on the utility of the approach with adults and ways in which fidelity can be achieved and the effectiveness of the intervention enhanced when working with an adult mental health client group. As mentioned in Chapter 9, Levels of Intervention, use of ASI requires specific post-graduate training to achieve the necessary certification.

Considering fidelity

The ASIFM (Parham et al., 2011) has two main sections, which relate to the structural and process elements of ASI. The structural elements section identifies different pieces of equipment that should be available; the level of training of the therapist; access to ongoing appropriate supervision; information that should be included within the assessment; and specifications for the environment (Schaaf & Mailloux, 2015). The process elements focus on therapeutic elements within the sessions, such as ensuring specific sensory experiences and development of a therapeutic relationship. The requirements for fidelity are well documented in Parham et al. (2011) and Schaaf and Mailloux's (2015) *Clinician's Guide for Implementing Ayres Sensory Integration®*, therefore the focus within this chapter will not be on detailing all of the specific components within this measure, but on identifying ways to meet criteria that are commonly thought to be more challenging within an adult mental health setting.

Structural elements of fidelity

Within the structural criteria of the ASIFM is a list of specific equipment that should be available within the setting, such as various types of swings, climbing equipment and gym balls (Parham et al., 2011; Schaaf & Mailloux, 2015). Several of the items tend to be beyond the scope of an adult mental health setting for reasons such as budget, space and risk. Also, very few adult mental health settings have a suitable room that could be transformed into a dedicated clinic space with multiple suspension points and storage for equipment. Suspension points in particular can be a non-negotiable feature in settings where risk of self-harm or ligatures is higher, making the use of specific swings not possible. In addition to this there is the barrier of equipment being of sufficient size for an adult, and where it is available, this also tends to significantly increase the cost. This is not an exhaustive list of the barriers, but in view of these barriers alone there can be a temptation to assume that this level of intervention is simply not achievable, or that sufficient fidelity cannot be achieved. However, the potential therapeutic benefits of this approach to an adult with sensory processing difficulties should not be discounted and a number of these barriers may be overcome through the creativity and adaptability of the therapist. While not an exhaustive list, ideas for how to begin doing so are provided below.

SWINGS

While it may not be possible to have a fixed point for a swing within the setting where you work there may be other ways to access similar opportunities. One could be within local parks with the types of swings available potentially varying in size, and type, such as two-point swings or basket swings. Use of these would need to be risk assessed for factors including weight and height, but there are parks that have swings of sufficient size to support an adult, and therefore this may be an option. Timing to avoid periods when a park is likely to be busy will also be an important consideration, and it is acknowledged that this may present additional challenges to accessing such opportunities. Therefore, for a number of people, identifying alternative ways to provide access to similar vestibular inputs may be the best option. Below are some possible ways to provide vestibular input that may not have the same intensity as a swing but could provide the most suitable substitute.

- Gym ball exercises such as bouncing on a gym ball will provide small amounts of linear vestibular input. Other options include activities that require the individual to roll forwards and backwards over the gym ball, perhaps while completing an activity or challenge involving grabbing or throwing items.

- Using a hammock may be an option in some settings or within someone's garden. This could be a way to provide slow, more controlled linear vestibular input.

- Body-weight exercises, for example a seesaw plank where you rock forwards and back, or burpees could provide more intense and variable vestibular input and challenge.

- Scooter boards. These can be obtained in adult sizes although at a higher cost. They can be useful for providing linear or rotary vestibular input, depending on the activity and direction of movement.

- Rowing machines provide linear vestibular input combined with proprioceptive input from the resistance, so may be a better option when needing to regulate responsivity to vestibular input or carefully consider the impact on arousal levels.

- Green gym equipment may be available within your local park and can include options such as rowers, cross trainers and pull-up bars. Outdoor gym equipment tends to be more freely moving, and can therefore provide faster vestibular input and more of a challenge to balance and maintain one's body position.

OTHER EQUIPMENT THAT CAN BE USEFUL FOR ADULT ASI SESSIONS

- Air beds/mattresses can be used for walking or crawling across to provide an added challenge for postural control and motor planning.

- Using a cross trainer provides linear vestibular input combined with proprioceptive input through both the arms and legs. It also requires coordinated movements and challenges postural control while in use.

- Weighted medicine balls provide a way to add weight into an activity in order to incorporate added proprioception or alter the level of challenge within a throwing and catching activity.

- Standing on a half balance ball or wobble board challenges postural control and balance in particular.
  - You can then increase the level of challenge further through activities such as passing a weighted ball or attempting to catch something while standing on it. Asking an individual to squat on it increases the challenge and also encourages increased proprioception.

- Suspension trainer. Various body-weight exercises such as press-ups or squats can be completed with these, which might help to increase the challenge or intensity of these exercises. They can be used to provide high levels of proprioception in particular, but also to vary levels of vestibular input through altering body position.

- Tactile boxes, which could contain items such as packing beads, sand or rice. To develop tactile discrimination, items can be hidden in the boxes. These can also challenge modulation of tactile input through the need to tolerate different textures.

- Peanut balls provide an alternative to a gym ball and can feel more stable to someone with poor postural control or who is gravitationally insecure.

- Play rolls are like a long gym ball and come in a variety of sizes, some of which are large enough for an adult. The benefit of this piece of equipment is that the shape and size enable you to sit on it at the same time as your client. This helps facilitate different sensory experiences and also collaborative engagement in challenges.

- Gym mats of a sufficient thickness to support safety are a necessary investment if you are going to be conducting ASI sessions.

- Dance sacks/body socks are large Lycra socks that are big enough for someone to climb inside. These are available in adult sizes and can be used to provide tactile input or resistance through pushing out against the sock once inside.

- Board games can be used to create a range of challenges within a session. To encourage linear movement and postural control you can play a game where you have to roll forwards over a peanut ball to reach and move the pieces each time. Locating pieces can provide a visual discrimination challenge.

- Bean bags can help to ensure safety by providing additional support to prevent a gym ball from moving or for cushioning if rolling over a ball.

- A whiteboard or blackboard can be helpful to map out ideas with a client at the beginning of a session, or to draw a target for use in different challenges and activities within the session.

USEFUL SMALLER ITEMS OF EQUIPMENT TO PROVIDE OPPORTUNITIES

- Craft materials such as clay, paint, pastels and chalk. These can be used to challenge both tactile modulation and discrimination through handling different textures, adjusting the grip required in response to the feel of the item, and tolerating residue left on the hands from the items.

- Shaving foam. Items can be concealed in the foam for the client to locate to develop tactile discrimination. Or an activity might be used that involves drawing in the foam to challenge tactile modulation.

- Sand pit/box. Items can be concealed within the sand, similar to shaving foam, or a client could be challenged to place their hand or foot into the sand, developing tactile modulation.

- Straws can be used for oral-motor activities such as blowing items around the room, for example air football. Oral motor activities can both provide effective regulation and also support development of postural control.

- A range of balls in different sizes, to create challenges and games for developing praxis skills and visual tracking.

- Cones can be used to increase the challenge of an activity through a requirement to navigate in and out of the cones. A game could include knocking down the cones as targets.

- Water beads can be used to challenge tactile modulation; they tend to be easier to tolerate than some materials so can be used effectively as a graded challenge.

ITEMS FOR CREATING A SAFE SPACE WITHIN SESSIONS

Where possible, provision of a 'safe space' that a client can access as needed during ASI sessions is advocated. During ASI sessions a therapist actively challenges the client, which has the potential to lead to periods where they become overloaded or in too high a state of arousal. Therefore, a space where they can retreat for periods to become more regulated is important. This space is sometimes known as a 'womb space' due to being an area designed to instil feelings of security and containment (Bundy & Szklut, 2020; Richter & Oetter, 1990). There is no exact recipe for this space, but the idea is for it to be low demand and create opportunities for deep pressure input. Wherever possible, this space should be created with your client. Items that may be helpful within this space include:

- bean bags and cushions
- soft blankets
- massage tools
- scented items
- items from a sensory kit or box if they have one.

Process elements of fidelity

The ASIFM includes ten process elements relating to: physical safety; type of sensory opportunities; sensory modulation; challenging postural, ocular, oral or bilateral motor control; praxis; collaboration; providing the 'just right challenge'; ensuring success; engagement through play; and the therapeutic alliance (Parham et al., 2011; Schaaf & Mailloux, 2015). Miller and Parham (2020) describe these elements as capturing both the 'art and science of therapy' as they guide the therapist in how to implement the theory of ASI within sessions. Some of these elements translate naturally to working with an adult client group, particularly within mental health, where development of a therapeutic alliance and identifying the just right challenge are key in most interventions. However, there are also process elements that therapists tend to identify as providing increased challenge when working with adults, particularly the criteria relating to playfulness and collaboration, and supporting the client to take the lead within the session. Play does not immediately seem relevant to an adult client group and can be too easily dismissed by some therapists as an element of fidelity that cannot be achieved, or that is only relevant when working with children. While collaboration with clients is central to practice in mental health, it is the specific nuances to ASI that can be more of a challenge. Collaboration in ASI entails the therapist presenting opportunities but with the direction of the session being led by the client (Bundy & Szklut, 2020). When working with adult clients, especially when attempting to engage in a new unfamiliar therapy, reaching the point where they begin to direct the session can be more of a challenge than with a naturally curious and playful child. These two aspects of fidelity will be considered further below.

PLAYFULNESS

Play is a word that is often associated with children, and rightly so, as it is a key occupation of childhood and development (Lynch & Moore, 2016). As a result, the relevance to an adult client group can be missed, and play can be seen as something that is not age appropriate, leading to this aspect of fidelity being too readily dismissed. However, evoking a sense of playfulness in adults has been suggested to help alter their approach to situations, develop problem-solving, and support them in being willing to accept the potential for failure in activities (Guitard et al., 2005). It has also been suggested to support the development of adaptive responses to stress (Clifford et al., 2024). Therefore, this could be an important component of intervention in an adult mental health setting. In addition, a number of the adults who are under adult mental health services may have had difficult childhoods and potentially decreased opportunities for play as a child, therefore missing an important developmental experience (Allee-Herndon et al., 2019). As highlighted earlier, ASI has a strong developmental focus, and therefore incorporating playful opportunities for an adult who may not have had these in their own childhood could hold increased value in the therapeutic process. For others it may provide a sense of reminiscing on positive childhood experiences that could facilitate more active engagement within the session. Engaging in a playful interaction can also shift the felt power dynamic between therapist and client towards a more collaborative approach, which is an important component of ASI sessions. These are just a few reasons the importance of this aspect within ASI should not be dismissed.

In considering this aspect of fidelity we perhaps need to begin with reframing our understanding of play and how this may be incorporated into sessions.

While play for a child often involves toys or games this does not need to be the case for adults. Beginning by considering the occupations we replace play with as we age is a helpful starting point. For adults, activities that are playful often involve an element of competition with others and this can be a useful aspect to add into ASI sessions to more fully engage your client. This is one way in which when engaging an adult in play you will need to be much more active than when doing so with a child, in order to facilitate that playfulness. Consider ways in which you can create a sense of competition in the activities within the session. This could be done by trying to complete more of a particular exercise than the other, activities that involve aiming at a target, using games such as Jenga or racing to locate an item. You will need to develop your own sense of creativity and improvisation to achieve this aspect, but it is important to do so.

Another element of play in ASI sessions with children is theming the sessions in connection with a character or game they like to increase engagement and facilitate imagination (Schaaf & Maillloux, 2015). When working with adults this can be harder to do but there are ways it can still be achieved. One way to do this may be to consider game shows or reality shows they watch, and consider whether there are elements that can be integrated into sessions to support engagement in a game or challenge. Consider if their preferred show can be used to spark ideas and creativity within what you are doing.

Playfulness could also be seen as promoting a sense of creativity through engagement in activities that provide a freedom in what they create or produce. Consider how you could use an art-based activity to enable a sense of playfulness. Think of activities such as creating a picture on a giant piece of paper across the floor with different materials that may also provide a range of tactile experiences. This could also be done by arranging different items around the room to create an image, which may also support opportunities for motor planning and movement within the process. There are a number of potential ways in which this element can be achieved, and these are a few ideas and suggestions to help you begin to consider how to implement this element of fidelity in your sessions.

COLLABORATION AND ENCOURAGING CLIENT-LED ACTIVITIES

Reaching the point where your client begins to take more of a lead within an ASI session can be challenging when working with adults, for a number of reasons. Adults within mental health are often used to engaging in predominantly therapist-led therapies where there is a set structure, or they are responding to therapist directions or questions. While as a therapist using ASI you are guiding the session, the format often feels much more open and can be slightly overwhelming at first for the client. For this reason, although your early ASI sessions with an adult are likely to be more led by you, the aim will be for you to gradually step back. Below are some suggestions for ways in which you can facilitate this process.

- Bring a range of items into the session to spark ideas. Having the visual cues may spark thoughts or memories that could support development of ideas.

- Use a board at the beginning of the session to map out possible ideas together, creating an overall list. Ask your client to then select what to do next from the board.

- Take turns in suggesting what to do next to gradually shift responsibility to the client.

- You as the therapist might decide the overall activity, but the client then decides how it will be completed, or specific challenges within the activity.

- Ask the client to help you set up for the session. This provides them with the opportunity to arrange the room and put out equipment of their choice, which may encourage them to direct the session to a greater extent.

Reaching the point where the client begins to actively direct the session may take time and a number of sessions, but they are likely to gradually adjust to the process and different way of working. The altered power dynamic and ability to self-direct is not only of importance in relation to fidelity but will also hold added value to a client within an adult mental health setting who experiences limited autonomy in other areas.

Identifying suitable spaces

Finding a dedicated space to conduct ASI sessions is a common challenge within mental health settings. One reason is that in order to conduct sessions safely and enable a range of opportunities for movement, there is a need for sufficient space, which is not often readily available. Many therapists use a multi-purpose activity space or a room in a client's home to conduct the intervention sessions which, while not ideal, can be adapted to meet need. Examples of spaces that tend to be used include a gym room, activity room, garden area, green spaces such as a park, play parks and a client's living room, but there are likely to be many more options.

When identifying where to conduct your sessions some of the factors you will need to consider include the affordances it provides; opportunities for sensations and free movement around the space; accessibility; and ability to manage risks within the space as needed. Using a non-clinic space has added challenges and is likely to require increased planning and preparation on your part as a therapist. To ensure you are best prepared and able to make best use of the space to achieve your client's therapeutic goals, a helpful strategy is to complete an audit of the space you intend to use, to review and identify how it can best be used, and what you need to consider when using that space. To help you do this an ASI planning template is provided at the end of this chapter, along with completed examples for a park space and a garden area.

Whatever space you choose to use, planning is going to be key, and an important factor in supporting the success of your sessions through best enabling you to meet your client's needs. ASI is an individually tailored and evolving intervention process (Schaaf & Mailloux, 2015) and that reactive adaptation and adjustment needed by the therapist can only be best achieved through a strong knowledge of ASI principles, a thorough assessment of client needs, and an active awareness of the affordances of the environment where your sessions take place.

Mentoring

Engagement in mentoring is a requirement of formal training in the use of ASI and strongly advocated by Schaaf and Mailloux in their clinician's guide to using the approach (2015). This is perhaps of even greater importance when working with an adult mental health client group where use of the approach is very much evolving and requires increased creativity and adaptation to achieve the requirements of fidelity. The purpose of such sessions should be to support reflection on your overall development as an ASI practitioner, and also to promote reflection on sessions completed with specific clients. Having a mentor observe a session where possible is also an invaluable learning opportunity to enable focused feedback and encourage alternative ways of thinking and responding within your sessions. Ideally, where possible it is helpful if that mentor has similar clinical experience, but there are also benefits to accessing sessions with a mentor from a different clinical setting who may ask you to explain your reasoning to a greater extent and challenge you to consider approaches that you may not immediately consider using with your client group.

Engagement in some form of group supervision or peer supervision is also likely to be highly valuable when working with an adult client group. As discussed above, there are particular challenges apparent when working with adults, and therefore reflecting on and sharing ideas with others working in a similar way and with similar resources is likely to be of great use in enabling you to develop your approach further.

Summary
While completing ASI intervention with an adult that adheres to fidelity carries added complexities, that does not mean it cannot be achieved. Not all clients will require this level of intervention, but for those that do, it is important to consider how to adapt your intervention to ensure it remains client-centred, focused on their specific sensory processing challenges, and reactive to their needs and goals. Engaging a client in this level of intervention will require creativity and adaptability on your part, which can be supported through engagement in mentoring and peer support sessions.

ASI® space planning template

Space identified:

Access considerations Examples include opening times, busy periods, proximity to client's address, other people accessing the space		
Item or equipment Depending on the space, this could be already available or items that can be taken into the space	**Opportunities provided** Consider sensations, opportunities for praxis, postural control and grading	**Risk considerations** e.g. weight restrictions, safety checks needed & frequency
1.		
2.		
3.		
4.		
5.		
6.		
7.		
8.		
9.		
10.		

★

Example completed forms

These are generalized ideas only and are likely to be more detailed when assessing a specific setting known to you.

Space identified: Play park		
Access considerations	Quieter times likely to include during school hours/term time.	
	Potential for variable/unsteady surfaces.	
Item or equipment	**Opportunities provided**	**Risk considerations**
Swings	Depending on the type of swing, could provide linear or rotary vestibular input; pushing someone else on the swing could provide proprioceptive input.	Particular risk considerations for this environment are likely to include the weight restrictions and size of different items of equipment. There are play parks that have a greater range of swings, some of which can support a greater weight range, but it is advisable to carefully risk assess prior to visiting with a client.
Balance beams	Challenges vestibular processing and balance; motor planning to determine how to successfully navigate the route across the beams.	
Zip wires	Provides intense linear vestibular input; challenges maintenance of postural control; motor planning in preparing to push off and successfully complete the action.	Consider the surfaces below the equipment and what materials have been used to promote safety. Checks for wear and tear may be completed by those who maintain the grounds, but as the frequency of this will not be known to you it is advisable to complete visual checks of the equipment prior to each session.
Roundabouts	Provides opportunities for rotary vestibular input, motor planning through turning and spinning the roundabout.	
Sand pit	Challenges ability to tolerate different textures if on bare skin, walking on different surfaces provides opportunities for motor planning and vestibular input.	Impact of weather on safety needs to be considered, e.g. equipment more slippery when raining.
Hanging bars	Could be used for pull-up motions to provide proprioceptive input or swinging along the bars to also gain vestibular input.	

cont.

Space identified:	Garden or green open space
Access considerations	If a shared green space, access by others will need to be considered.
	Different levels or varied surfaces within a garden space may increase accessibility considerations.

Item or equipment	Opportunities provided	Risk considerations
Flower beds/pots	Challenges postural control through bending down/leaning over; level of challenge can be altered by using raised beds or flower beds; development of tactile modulation through tolerating with or without gloves; proprioceptive input from digging holes or digging up weeds; required bilateral skills in completing these tasks.	The primary risk considerations in this type of environment will include any physical limitations relevant to your client. These could result from a health condition, or their weight, mobility and physical fitness. You will also need to consider being appropriately dressed, including suitable footwear for the different surfaces and clothing that allows freedom to move and bend. Other relevant considerations include an individual's risk profile such as self-harm or aggression towards others and how items within the environment or that will be taken into the environment could increase these risks.
Different surfaces, e.g. grass, soil, pebbles	Challenges postural control changing from one surface to another; variation between shoes on and off to challenge tactile modulation.	
Conkers, leaves, horse chestnuts	Collecting these could provide varying tactile challenges; spotting and identifying the items could also be used to develop visual discrimination. Level of challenges could also be increased through moving over different surfaces in order to reach the items.	
Soil	Digging and moving the soil provides proprioceptive and vestibular input; also challenges motor planning to complete the task effectively.	

CONCLUSION/KEY LEARNING

Ayres Sensory Integration has potential applicability across the life span, including for clients with mental health needs. This chapter provides ideas for adapting items and spaces in view of risk and age appropriateness.

Key points

- Use of ASI with this client group will require creativity and adaptability on the part of the therapist.
- All aspects of fidelity remain relevant across the life span but may be implemented in different ways.

CHAPTER 13

Outcome Measurement

REBECCA MATSON

Outcome measurement is an important part of our practice to ensure we can identify whether a client's goals have been achieved; the approach used has been effective; and to identify any changes needed moving forwards. It is also a requirement of our professional standards as occupational therapists (RCOT, 2021). Outcome measurement should inform both our approach in working with individuals and also our overall approach to the service we provide, as part of evidence-based practice and providing the best possible care to those we work with (Breckenridge & Jones, 2015; Duncan & Murray, 2012).

While sensory approaches are a bottom-up approach, the goals we agree with our clients should relate to the functional or occupational aim they want to achieve, and that is likely to be facilitated by intervention focused on altering their underlying sensory responses or impairments in processing. Sensory processing differences only become a problem when they prevent us from doing what we want to or need to be able to do and that is why it is important we consider them in this context. Having a clear occupational goal also creates a meaningful and shared understanding of the overall aim of intervention.

Therefore, the first stage in ensuring adequate outcome measurement needs to happen earlier on as part of your assessment process. If a measure has not been completed at this early assessment stage, then it cannot be used to inform outcome measurement as it will not be able to capture change, but only current performance. An important factor to consider when assessing need should therefore be whether these measures are not only effective in capturing someone's baseline but also valid and reliable if readministered following a period of intervention.

Schaaf and Mailloux (2015) advocate for the setting of proximal and distal goals in sensory interventions; the proximal goal is focused on capturing underlying sensory or motor changes and the distal goal on capturing the overall occupational or functional goal. The two however should be connected and not fully stand-alone goals. When written well, the proximal and distal goals combined should help illustrate how those underlying changes will enable your client to achieve their overall goal and therefore more fully demonstrate the value of the intervention. They will also provide a shared understanding with your client of the benefits and value of facilitating those underlying changes, and are likely to gain increased investment in agreed interventions. In view of this connection, capturing changes in both the underlying components and the overall occupational goal is highly important, and consideration needs to be given to including outcome measures for each of these aspects. If either component is not measured, then how can you demonstrate that the occupational gains are the result of your intervention?

Within this chapter both the factors to be considered when choosing suitable outcome measures, and potential choices for these, will be discussed to support you as a therapist in identifying which may be of benefit within your practice. Further details are available on the use of each of the sensory assessments discussed below in Chapter 8, Assessment and Goal Setting.

Capturing sensory changes

When measuring changes in sensory processing there are several factors that need to be considered and that may influence your choice. Often, the choice can be made from routine or availability alone without considering effectiveness or suitability to a sufficient degree. While it may take negotiation and investment in additional resources, obtaining tools that best enable you to evidence the effectiveness of therapy will be of inherent value to your practice. Within this chapter a few potential choices will be discussed which, while not exhaustive, are perhaps the best current validated measures for this purpose. The Adolescent/Adult Sensory Profile (Brown & Dunn, 2002) is not included within this section as according to Brown (2020) test–retest reliability is yet to be evaluated for this measure.

Adult/Adolescent Sensory History (ASH) (May-Benson, 2015)

The ASH is one of the more comprehensive measures of sensory processing available for use with adults, which therefore may make it a good choice for outcome measurement. It has been suggested to have strong test stability and test–retest reliability, which May-Benson and Easterbrooks-Dick (2016) assert makes the assessment suitable to measure change, though they do not explicitly state if it is intended to be used in outcome measurement. One area of caution is the nature of a self-reporting assessment such as this, and the potential impact of that on readministration. As engagement in sensory interventions should lead to an individual's awareness of their sensory processing increasing, this may inadvertently lead to a decline or lack of change in scores following intervention not due to a lack of progress, but due to an increased understanding and therefore increased ability to reflect on and identify their sensory responses. This is not to say that this tool should not be used in this way, but that it may be advisable to use another form of assessment alongside to verify changes more fully.

Sensory Processing Measure, Second Edition (SPM-2) (Parham et al., 2021)

The SPM-2 is an updated version of the original Sensory Processing Measure with the difference that there are now forms validated for use with a wider population, which includes four months up to 87 years of age, which therefore have potential for use with the adult mental health population. The SPM-2 has been found to have good overall test–retest reliability and criterion-related validity (Parham et al., 2021), and therefore is likely to support an accurate assessment and is a potentially useful outcome measurement. As yet, however, a lack of data is available in relation to responsiveness and all participants within the validation of the tool were from within the United States, which may impact on reliability with populations outside of this. It should also be noted that Parham et al. (2021) do not identify whether the tool is suitable or intended for use as an outcome measure and therefore caution may be needed when using in this way (Brown et al., 2023). As with the ASH, due to this being a self-report measure, there is a risk of answers being influenced by familiarity with the questions when readministered and the person being more aware of the impact of any sensory processing difficulties following the intervention process. This could potentially lead to some over-reporting of symptoms and as a result it may not fully capture improvements in the different areas. One way to potentially counter the impact of this could be to use both the self-report and an observer version to gain differing views on progress. Parham et al. (2021) suggest that this tool should not be used in isolation, and this therefore may also apply to outcome measurement and the need for an additional way of capturing changes in sensory processing.

Sensory Integration and Praxis Test (SIPT) (Ayres, 1989) or the Evaluation in Ayres Sensory Integration (EASI) (Mailloux et al., 2018)

While neither the SIPT nor EASI are validated for use with adults at the time of writing, they may well be a useful way of obtaining clinical observations in relation to specific areas of challenge and to identify if there has been an improvement in these areas. Due to the lack of validation for adults, and to minimize demands on the client, it may be best to solely repeat the sub-tests that identified areas of concern. While the recommendation is for these only to be used for more qualitative observations, it would still be advisable to keep to recommended time periods for readministration when using them to support outcome measurement. Sub-tests from one of these assessments may be useful to support or challenge scores from a readministered self-report assessment such as the SPM-2 or ASH and provide a fuller picture in relation to any progress made, the added complexity being that interpretation will be much more dependent upon therapist knowledge and skill due to being utilized outside of standardization.

Clinical observations

There are various versions of clinical observations, some of which are freely available and others that have supporting guidance, such as Blanche et al. (2020), making them a fairly accessible option for outcome measurement. As administering clinical observations would not provide a numerical measure of change, they may not be best suited to a standalone outcome measure, but could be used to corroborate changes suggested through other measures or to provide further information in relation to the specific improvements in sensory processing. Certain clinical observations can be chosen to measure the areas of priority identified within the initial goals for intervention rather than readministration of all clinical observations initially used, to allow for a more focused and lower-demand re-assessment process for the client.

Capturing occupational changes

As noted above, as occupational therapists it is important that improvements in occupational performance and functioning are noted and measured alongside any improvements in sensory processing. When choosing which outcome measure to use there are a range of important factors, such as what the overall goals for intervention are and how they can best be captured; what measures are validated for the client group; reliability of the measure in capturing change;

and time demands of the assessment both in view of potential workload as a therapist and the demands of the assessment process on the client. The potential outcome measures below are not exhaustive but should give a useful starting point in deciding which to use in each case. For further general guidance in relation to choosing outcome measures, a guidance document is available through the Royal College of Speech and Language Therapists (2019), entitled *Key Questions to Ask When Selecting Outcome Measures: A Checklist for Allied Health Professionals*, which was developed in partnership with various professional bodies including the Royal College of Occupational Therapists.

Goal attainment scaling (GAS) (Kiresuk et al., 1994)

Goal attainment scaling (GAS) is perhaps one of the outcome measures most frequently connected to sensory-based interventions in practice, with its use being apparent in several studies and advocated in resources such as Schaaf and Mailloux's clinician's guide (Schaaf & Mailloux, 2015). While its use has become more commonly associated with paediatric interventions, GAS originated in mental health as a way of capturing change that was perhaps not easily quantifiable (Kiresuk & Sherman, 1968). Another benefit of this measure is it allows individualized goals to be scaled rather than the measuring of pre-determined factors, and therefore is often considered more person-centred (Logan et al., 2022). Kings College London provide a few freely available resources to support clinician use of GAS in practice.[1]

However, as GAS relies on the rating of individualized goals, the reliability of the measure is dependent on how well the initial goals are set and scaled. A GAS goal is scaled according to an expected outcome of between -2 and +2 (Turner-Stokes, 2009). A therapist starts by agreeing a baseline of performance with the client which forms -1 on the scale. 0 reflects the expected outcome of intervention, with +1 and +2 reflecting greater than anticipated change and -1 and -2 reflecting less than expected change. The difference between the levels should be in equal increments to support reliability of the measure, which can create a challenge (Turner-Stokes, 2009). GAS also requires the identification of a quantifiable factor that can be measured to allow scaling, such as the time in which someone will be able to complete a task; the number of verbal prompts that will be needed; or the level of support with which they will be able to complete a task. As GAS is used to capture changes in a client-centred goal, the goal may not always lend itself to capturing such factors. It is worth making

---

1 Accessible at www.kcl.ac.uk/cicelysaunders/resources

this initial time investment to achieve a clear goal to support later reliability in outcome measurement.

GAS goals often focus on a specific component of an overarching goal, or a short-term goal that helps work towards a longer-term goal. As with any goal, the relevance of this goal is dependent on the meaning or purpose for that individual. Below is an example of a scaled goal for an individual, Laura, who is struggling to attend the ward cooking group due to gradually becoming overwhelmed by the level of sensory stimulation in the session. This goal could be part of an overall goal an individual has in relation to developing their cooking skills or engaging in more activities with other people, for example. There could be a whole range of reasons for choosing to scale this activity and the factor of time, but the important point is to be sure on why it is you are scaling that particular factor and why it is relevant in capturing progress towards their goal. Currently Laura is managing to attend and participate in the group for up to 15 minutes before becoming too agitated and leaving the session. The overall aim is for her to participate in the full session, but the outcome will be rated on gradual increments towards this to acknowledge her progression.

Goal: For Laura to participate in the cooking group for the whole session (60 minutes)	
Current performance: Laura participates in the group for up to 15 minutes before leaving	
+2	Laura participates in the group for 60 minutes
+1	Laura participates in the group for 45 minutes
0	Laura participates in the group for 30 minutes
-1	Laura participates in the group for 15 minutes
-2	Laura does not participate in the group

Whichever element of a goal is chosen for scaling, ensure this relates to a priority for that individual and what they want to be able to achieve as an outcome. While one person may want to be able to engage in activity for a longer period of time or more often, another may be more concerned with increasing their independence within that activity or the number of activities they engage in. Identifying their priorities will help motivate progress towards the goal and investment in the process of sensory interventions to help them achieve it.

Model of Human Occupation Screening Tool (MOHOST) (Parkinson et al., 2006)

The Model of Human Occupation Screening Tool (MOHOST) is designed to measure occupational performance in relation to six main areas or components: motivation for occupation, pattern of occupation, communication and interaction, process skills, motor skills, and an individual's environment (Parkinson et al., 2006). These factors are evaluated according to a FAIR rating scale based upon whether a factor facilitates (F), allows (A), inhibits (I) or restricts (R) occupational participation (Parkinson et al., 2006). The MOHOST has been identified as a reliable assessment tool with a range of client groups and has been suggested to be easy to use and helpful in guiding the setting or goals and identified intervention (Bugajska & Brooks, 2021). It has also been acknowledged as an occupationally focused outcome measure that can be useful in capturing change in mental health populations (Kirsh et al., 2019; Kramer et al., 2009). One reservation suggested is that the ability to capture change can be dependent on the severity of the mental health condition and that it is not sufficiently sensitive to capture smaller levels of change or progress (Bugajska & Brooks, 2021).

An added potential benefit, perhaps, when using the MOHOST in connection with sensory interventions is that the measure considers motor and process skills in the context of occupation and therefore may more easily show a correlation to measures used to capture sensory processing changes. Consideration should, however, be given to factors such as length of time between administrations and the impact this may have on the level of change as well as the objectivity of the therapist. As this is an observational assessment it may be subject to bias on the part of the therapist, and is likely to benefit from the input of further therapists, staff members and the client themselves when administering both at baseline and at the point of outcome measurement. As it is therapist completed rather than self-report, however, that does reduce assessment load for the client themselves.

Occupational Self-Assessment (OSA) (Baron et al., 2006)

The Occupational Self-Assessment (OSA) is a self-report assessment designed to actively support goal setting through the identification of occupational performance in a range of areas, and guide connected prioritization of the areas considered most important by the client (Kielhofner et al., 2010). Each of these areas is rated against a four-point scale which therefore allows for identification of self-perceived progress when readministered (Baron et al., 2006). The OSA has been found to be sensitive in capturing change over time in different areas of occupational performance, which may therefore make it a suitable choice for outcome measurement (Kielhofner et al., 2010). It is also relatively quick to administer, which is perhaps more important in sensory interventions where there is also the need to measure sensory changes, therefore increasing potential demands on the therapist and the client.

The OSA is based on pre-determined areas of occupational performance which are therefore broader in nature and could be less likely to capture an individual's primary concerns than the GAS. It may therefore also take more effort on the part of the therapist to demonstrate the connection between areas on the assessment and underlying performance components such as sensory processing. A significant benefit, however, is the prioritization of areas guided by the tool, which ensures that is a central feature of assessment and outcome measurement.

Model of Human Occupation Exploratory Level Outcome Ratings (MOHO-ExpLOR) (Cooper et al., 2018; Parkinson et al., 2014)

The Model of Human Occupation Exploratory Level Outcome Ratings (MOHO-ExpLOR) was developed as an alternative to the MOHOST assessment in response to critiques that the MOHOST was not sensitive enough to change for those in a more severe or more acute period of illness or where progress may be impacted by cognitive deficits (Bugajska & Brooks, 2021). Similar to the MOHOST, the MOHO-ExpLOR is a therapist-rated tool but where the gathering of information from various sources is encouraged to support the assessment process and ratings. The tool, however, places increased emphasis on measuring the impact of a client's environment upon occupational performance, with ten of the items measured focusing on personal factors and ten focusing on their environment (Parkinson et al., 2014).

There is a lack of published studies into the use of the MOHO-ExpLOR as yet, but the identified increased sensitivity to change may be of particular benefit when working with clients with more chronic conditions. When sensory processing challenges are identified in adulthood they have often been present for a prolonged time and may have led to more compounded difficulties due to the absence of intervention in this particular area. Change resulting from intervention can therefore also appear slower and may be better captured by a tool that has increased sensitivity to change in different areas of functioning.

Canadian Occupational Performance Measure (COPM) (Law et al., 1994a, 1998)

The Canadian Occupational Performance Measure (COPM) is a self-report assessment and outcome measure designed to support evaluation of occupational performance in relation to the areas of self-care, productivity and leisure. A benefit is that it is suitable for use across the life span and with a range of client groups (Law et al., 1994a). Similar to the OSA, it is designed to support goal setting and prioritization of the most important areas for intervention. The COPM has been found to have an acceptable level of reliability and internal consistency (Bosch, 1995; Sanford et al., 1994) and to be responsive to change in occupational performance, suggesting a good potential utility as an outcome measure (Law et al., 1994b). Overall a need for a higher level of validation has been identified to verify these properties particularly in terms of criterion validity (Ohno et al., 2021).

A particular benefit of the COPM that has been highlighted within research is the potential to support goals for measurement that are more client-centred, rather than the therapist's perception of what they consider important for that person (Richard & Knis-Matthews, 2010). The COPM has also been used within the literature as an outcome measure in studies relating to sensory integration, but primarily with child client groups (Stackhouse et al., 2023), and has not been as widely adopted within adult mental health settings.

Quality of life measures

Another potential way to measure changes when carrying out sensory interventions is through the use of quality of life measures. A number of these are freely available and are often relatively low demand to complete, which could be of benefit when also completing sensory assessments with a client. It is beyond the scope of this book to outline all possible quality of life measures that could be used, therefore focus will be given to a couple of examples that may be of use within mental health settings.

World Health Organization Quality of Life: WHOQOL-100 and WHOQOL-BREF

One potential quality of life measure is the WHOQOL-100, or the abbreviated version, the WHOQOL-BREF. The WHOQOL was designed to broaden the focus of outcome measurement beyond more medicalized aspects, such as absence of impairment, to consider an individual's overall life and different aspects within that, such as activities of daily life, social factors and level of independence (World Health Organization (WHO), 2012). The WHOQOL is available in a range of languages and the assessment and supporting manuals are free to download from the World Health Organization website. The full version of the WHOQOL consists of 100 self-rated questions using a Likert scale and focused on physical health, psychological health, social relationships and environment (WHO, 2012). The WHOQOL-BREF is reduced to 26 questions and therefore may be more suitable for working with clients where concentration may be an issue or there is a need to reduce demands in the assessments completed.

The 36-Item Short Form Survey Instrument (SF-36) (Ware & Sherbourne, 1992)

Another potential quality of life measure is the 36-Item Short Form Survey Instrument (SF-36) (Ware & Sherbourne, 1992), and is freely available for use through RAND, a not-for-profit research organization. The SF-36 includes 36 questions intended to measure self-evaluated physical functioning, roles, pain, general health, social functioning and mental health. As well as being frequently used in a range of practice settings it has also been used in a high number of research studies focusing on a range of populations (Lins & Carvalho, 2016). The measure is relatively quick to complete and to readminister, has been used with mental health populations including those with schizophrenia (Su et al., 2014), and has been found to be sensitive to change within mental health client groups overall (de Beurs et al., 2022).[2]

Warwick–Edinburgh Mental Wellbeing Scale (WEMWBS) (Tennant et al., 2007)

Depending on the areas of change identified as priorities, the Warwick–Edinburgh Mental Wellbeing Scale (WEMWBS) (Tennant et al., 2007) may also be a useful tool for outcome measurement. The difference with this tool is the focus solely on mental wellbeing rather than broader health. This is another relatively quick measure to complete, and has both a 14-question and a 7-question version available, both requiring Likert scale-style responses. The scale is free to use but you are required to first register for a licence identifying the intended usage.

Assessments of mental state or mood

As sensory processing impacts on our arousal levels and regulation, another way to capture positive changes as a result of sensory-based interventions could be through the use of psychometric assessments designed to measure factors such as anxiety levels or mood.

---

[2] Instructions on scoring the assessment can be found at www.rand.org/health-care/surveys_tools/mos/36-item-short-form/scoring.html

Generalized Anxiety Disorder Questionnaire (GAD-7) (Spitzer et al., 2006)

The Generalized Anxiety Disorder Questionnaire (GAD-7) is a free-to-use seven-item assessment designed to measure the prevalence of anxiety symptoms. The scale is short and quick to complete, so when used alongside other assessments will not place high additional demands on an individual. In response to each of the questions individuals rate how frequently they experienced different symptoms over the preceding two-week period to obtain an overall score. The GAD-7 is widely used in mental health practice and has been found sufficiently sensitive to capture change over time in response to interventions (Toussaint et al., 2020).

Hospital Anxiety and Depression Scale (HADS) (Zigmund & Snaith, 1983)

The Hospital Anxiety and Depression Scale (HADS) measures levels of both anxiety and depression through a self-report questionnaire consisting of 14 questions. Individuals are asked to rate their symptoms over the previous week from 0 to 3. The HADS is considered to be sensitive to change and therefore could be of use in showing changes in mood during sensory-based interventions. The ability to use this assessment as frequently as weekly makes it particularly useful for capturing gradual changes and could help a therapist track whether, for example, introducing a particular strategy is likely to have led to a shift in symptoms.

Sleep scales

Another option for a factor to measure is sleep patterns or quality. Sleep is an area that is often impacted in mental health conditions, and also in connection with sensory processing differences, so this may be a relevant factor to measure in connection with sensory interventions for your client group. One choice for measuring changes in sleep could be to use a sleep diary such as the one available from the Sleep Foundation (Sleep Foundation, 2023), which asks someone to record factors such as the number of times they woke in the night and how long they slept overall. Completion of a sleep diary may provide a more accurate picture if completed daily, but is reliant on this being done regularly. There are also assessments available to measure the quality of sleep, including the Pittsburgh Sleep Quality Index (Buysse et al., 1989), which is a self-report assessment likely to take around 5–10 minutes to complete. This is potentially lower demand than a sleep diary but as it asks someone to reflect on their sleep for the last month will be subject to the reliability of their recall over a longer period.

Reflective tools

The use of a reflective tool as part of the outcome measurement process can be an important part of your own evaluation both of their progress and of your own skill as a therapist. Reflecting on the process as a whole or specific sessions is important in considering potential factors in progress a client may have made, or also perhaps why an intervention has not achieved the desired effect. When using higher levels of sensory intervention, such as Ayres Sensory Integration, this can also be an important part of considering adherence to fidelity and therapist skill. Due to the nature of ASI sessions, as a therapist it can be difficult to achieve depth of reflection while in the session due to the need to be responsive to the client's lead and often being an active participant. Therefore ongoing reflections throughout and at the end of the intervention process can be invaluable.

In order to support this process a more widely used reflective tool could be utilized, such as Gibbs' reflective model (Gibbs, 1988), which is commonly used in healthcare practice as a whole. However, in order to increase the depth of reflection on specific sensory aspects of the session, it may be helpful to either also use, or replace this with, a tool such as the OTA–Watertown Clinical Assessment Worksheet, available as Appendix 12B in Windsor et al. (2001), which could support consideration of different aspects of sessions and a client's response to them, in order to review whether they achieved the intended outcome. An alternative to this, if completing ASI sessions, could be to self-rate the ASIFM following each session as a form of reflection on therapist performance and to guide alterations to future sessions.

CONCLUSION/KEY LEARNING

This chapter considers different approaches to outcome measurement in view of sensory processing, functioning and occupational performance.

Key points

- Measurement of both 'top-down' occupational factors and 'bottom-up' underlying components is needed to help evidence the effectiveness of sensory interventions.
- Outcome measurement should help evidence achievement of the goals set and should be informed by priority areas for the client and the service.

APPENDIX 1

Sensory Assessment Report Template

A blank version of this template can be downloaded from https://digitalhub.jkp.com/redeem using the code: KWSHBDS

Date: Name: Date of birth:

Assessor: Qualification:

Date(s) assessment completed:

Reason for referral

- Rationale provided for requesting a sensory assessment, including particular areas of concern, e.g. self-harming behaviours, social isolation.
- Any specific aims identified as desired outcomes from the assessment.

Presenting concerns

- Overview of any sensory concerns already identified, with examples of how they are seen day to day.
- Examples of how this is impacting on functioning.
- Any particularly problematic environments identified, e.g. certain areas of the ward or their work place.

Relevant historical information

- Information gathered as part of a review of records or background information prior to completing face-to-face assessment.

- Examples may include:
  - *premature birth or difficulties in delivery*
  - *developmental milestones*
  - *difficulties with schooling*
  - *early traumatic experiences*
  - *attachment experiences such as adoption.*

Assessments completed

Outline the assessment tools chosen, who completed them, a brief description of what they measure, and if they were completed in person or virtually.

e.g. Adult/Adolescent Sensory History (ASH) (May-Benson, 2015) completed on [DATE] by the service user themselves. This assessment considers sensory modulation, discrimination, postural-ocular skills, praxis and social-emotional functioning.

Summary of assessment findings

Sensory modulation

- Definition/description of sensory modulation.
- Depending on the number of difficulties within this area you may wish to discuss each sense separately or cluster certain senses together in relation to the impact of these difficulties, for example if the results of your assessment suggest difficulties with both visual and auditory modulation and the service user is struggling to access the local supermarket due to being overwhelmed by both of these aspects.
- Provide both examples drawn from the assessment questions, to help that person see how you have reached your conclusion, and examples from the information gathered in relation to their functioning that helps to confirm this area of difficulty.
- Outline if any senses are apparent strengths in relation to modulation that potentially could be used within the intervention process to support regulation.

Sensory discrimination

- Definition/description of sensory discrimination.
- Depending on the number of difficulties within this area you may wish to discuss each sense separately or cluster certain senses together in relation to the impact of these difficulties. For example, if the individual has identified

difficulties in relation to both tactile and proprioceptive discrimination, you may wish to draw a connection to the likely impact of this on motor skills.
- Provide both examples drawn from the assessment questions, to help that person see how you have reached your conclusion, and examples from the information gathered in relation to their functioning.
- Outline if any senses are apparent strengths in discrimination that potentially could be used within the intervention process to support information processing.

Motor planning/praxis and postural control

- Definition of praxis and the component parts of this.
- Examples drawn from the assessment questions or areas, to help that person see how you have reached your conclusion, but also examples from the information gathered in relation to their functioning.
- Discuss the connection of this to any difficulties identified in relation to discrimination or modulation.

Recommendations

- Within this section you should consider sensory strategies that may be beneficial, adaptations to the environment and suggested activities. Where specific guidance needs to be followed, for example weighted blanket guidance, ensure this is clearly stated and a link provided.
- You may also wish to include within this section recommendations in relation to suitable placements or living environments based upon the outcomes of the assessment. Recommendations may also inform approach to communication and interaction based upon sensory responses, e.g. maintaining a level tone of voice where auditory modulation is an issue.

Summary statement

This should be a short paragraph summarizing the main areas of difficulty identified through the assessment and, if relevant, may identify a particular pattern of difficulty, e.g. somatodyspraxia. Ensure you also define any such difficulties for the reader of the report.

Signature: Date:

For further information about this report please contact:

APPENDIX 2

Sensory Support Plan Template

A blank version of this template can be downloaded from https://digitalhub.jkp.com/redeem using the code: KWSHBDS

Name: Date:

Date for review:

Please contact for support in reviewing this plan:

My sensory preferences – what sensations do I respond well to and which ones are difficult for me?

Summary of sensations that are helpful and those that are problematic.

My sensory strategies – these strategies help me to feel more regulated and to engage in activities that are important to me

What is the item or activity?	When and where is it helpful?	Why should it be used?
Description of the item or activity. Pictures can be helpful.	Are there certain times when it is helpful or certain places where it is likely to be needed?	How would I or others know that I need to use the strategy?

★

Places and spaces – strategies for accessing places I need or want to go to

Place	What is difficult about it?	Strategy to support access, e.g. time of day, before or after certain activities

This plan should be reviewed in [X months] or following changes in the following:

Examples may include risk changes, e.g. self-harm, change of environment/placement, changes in mental health or physical health. List the factors most relevant to the person here.

★

APPENDIX 3

Sensory Group Programme

Preparing for the group

Rationale: This programme is designed to support individuals in developing awareness of their sensory needs and preferences in order to learn to use them more effectively and improve their self-regulation and wellbeing. Individuals do not need to have any identified sensory needs to benefit from this programme as we all use sensory strategies naturally within our daily lives, whether we are aware of it or not, and can all benefit from doing this more consciously. The focus of this group is on developing understanding of both arousal theory and sensory processing to enable individuals to be more regulated and support engagement in activities that they need to or want to do.

Participants: There is no set number of participants for this group, but it is likely to be most beneficial when there are enough participants to share ideas with each other, but not so many that it is difficult to express opinions or trial different strategies. Four to eight participants is a good group size for that reason.

Staffing: This will vary depending on setting but it is helpful to have two facilitators for this group where possible. This allows the facilitators to demonstrate differences in their own sensory preferences, and normalize the fact that we all have sensory preferences that are like part of our personality rather than a pathology. It also helps to monitor the reactions of group members to different strategies, such as autonomic reactions that may suggest they are feeling overwhelmed.

Location: A relaxed environment is helpful for this group to encourage group members to feel able to share. Therefore, it should contain features such as comfortable seating/different seating options so group members can choose according to preferences, sufficient space to trial strategies, and minimal distractions such as noise from a corridor.

★

Number of sessions: This group plan is separated into sessions, including an introductory session covering arousal levels and an introduction to the eight senses – taste, smell, auditory and visual input, touch, movement (vestibular and proprioceptive input) and interoception – and a final review session to summarize overall learning and develop individual sensory plans. Each session, lasting approximately 30 minutes, can be run separately week by week, or the sessions can be amalgamated into two longer sessions, for example. It would be advisable to avoid combining them further, such as into one day-long group, as this is likely to lead to sensory overload and impact on the potential benefits individuals may gain from trialling different strategies. You may wish to adjust the order of the sessions depending on your client group. For example, the sessions are ordered here to start with taste and smell as this is often a more accessible session, but if you are working with an eating disorders client group then it may be better to build towards rather than start with this session. Or if the group of people you are working with are quite active and interested in physical activity you may wish to start with the movement session to pique their interest and develop understanding.

Developing a sensory kit or plan: To support ongoing use of strategies participants should develop a sensory plan or kit as an outcome of the group. In order to do so it is important to have some way for participants to keep track of the strategies they trial and which ones they find helpful. This could be through using a checklist or perhaps adding to a sensory kit as they go through the sessions.

Session 1: How the senses impact on our arousal levels

Session aim: To better understand fluctuations in mood and how the senses impact on these.

Understanding arousal levels

Arousal levels relate to how calm or alert we feel. All of us experience fluctuations in our arousal levels during the day, and this can often happen before we are aware of it. Being able to manage our level of arousal is important to enable us to engage in the occupations that we need to or want to do. There are various models to help understand the impact of our arousal levels; perhaps one of the most helpful to explain this is Dan Siegel's Window of Tolerance (Siegel, 1999). It may be helpful to print out a diagram of this to refer to during this and future group sessions when helping group members to consider the impact of different strategies on their arousal levels.

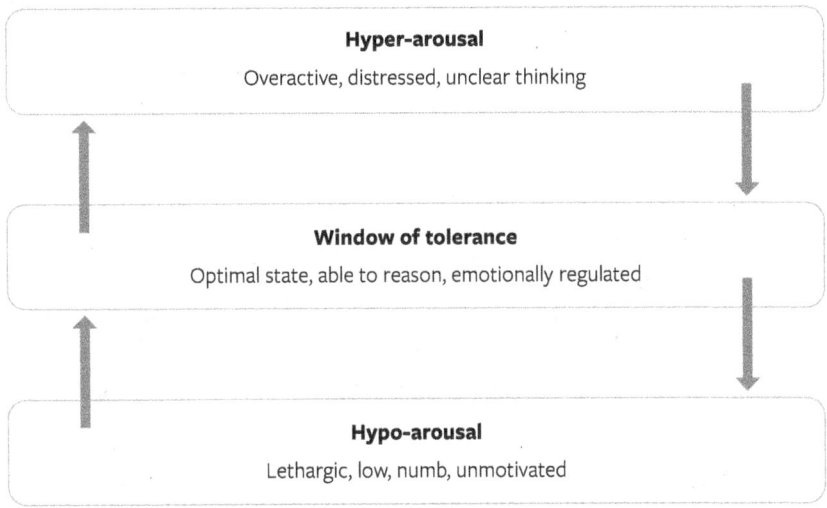

Figure A3.1 *Window of Tolerance (Siegel, 1999)*

Ask each group member to spend a bit of time making a note of what each of the levels looks like for them – what would they be doing, what would their mood be like, where would they be and how much might they be interacting with others? They do not need to share this with anyone else in the group but ask them to keep hold of it to look back on when considering times that different strategies may be useful and to help track their impact on their arousal levels.

Depending on what we want to do, it may be helpful to be in different states of arousal, therefore there is no one ideal state. For example, you will need to be in a much higher state of arousal for engaging in an aerobics class than when relaxing on a spa day. Sensory input can both affect our arousal level unintentionally due to the various inputs we take in throughout the day, and also be used consciously to alter our arousal state and help us to engage. The sensory inputs that affect us will vary from individual to individual, as will those that are helpful. During this group you will develop your understanding of your own sensory triggers, and sensory experiences that help you to feel more regulated. Think of how one person may feel energized when listening to live music by the level of noise, the beat of the music, and the people around them, while another person may quickly become overwhelmed by people bumping into them, the pulsing of the speakers and the different sounds.

It is important to remember during these sessions that there is no right or wrong response and to respect each other's reactions. Learning about our sensory preferences in a group allows us to learn from strategies others use and to appreciate the differences and similarities in our responses.

Activity: How am I feeling right now? Ask participants to reflect on where they are within their window of tolerance right now. What have they done so far that day that may have made them feel like that? What in the session might be making them feel like that? For example, did they make a hot drink to bring to the group?

Understanding our senses

Ask participants to identify the senses they are aware of. Most likely they will identify five senses, but if they have already completed some form of assessment or screening with you they may identify more. Discuss that within sensory strategies we will be thinking about eight senses: taste, smell, vision, hearing/sound, touch, proprioception, vestibular input and interoception.

Discuss that you will consider each sense in more depth over the coming sessions, but provide a brief explanation for now of the senses group members may be less familiar with. The list below may help with this:

- Proprioception: This relates to feedback from our muscles, and our sense of body position. Ask participants to clench their fists and release – discuss that the feeling of tension they felt going up their arms is proprioceptive feedback.

- Vestibular: This relates to our sense of gravity or balance, and our awareness of movement. Discuss that we activate this sense when we move our heads out of their central position; think about bending down to pick up something off the floor.

- Interoception: This relates to our awareness of internal sensations such as when we are hungry or thirsty, also how we feel emotionally in connection with that – for example, a churning stomach may reflect anxiety.

Discuss that everyone will already have sensory-based strategies that they use even if they are not conscious of them. Can they think of any examples? *Ideas could include drinking coffee to feel more alert, stroking a pet to feel calmer, sucking on a mint to help concentrate.*

Ask participants to try to notice and keep track over the following week of the different strategies they use, and when they use them, to start to understand the strategies that they already use.

End by summarizing the overall purpose of the group programme: to better understand their own sensory responses and to be able to use these more effectively to support their self-regulation. Through doing this the aim is for them to be able to use the strategies to help them do what they need to and want to do.

Group guidelines

It may be helpful at the end of this session to agree group guidelines or expectations for sessions amongst those who have attended. Now that group members have a better idea of the purpose of the group they are likely to be better able to do this. The type of expectations you may agree include common group expectations such as respect for each other's contributions but could also include others related to the group focus such as that group members are able to use strategies to self-regulate as needed throughout the sessions such as getting up and moving around or using different fidget items.

Taste and olfactory strategies
Items to bring to the session

For the session you should have a selection of the following:

- Oils or products in a variety of scents: Lavender, mint/peppermint, citrus scents such as lemon or orange, eucalyptus, a floral scent such as geranium or rose, vanilla.
- Suggested types of products: Shower gel, hand creams, scented sprays, aromatherapy oils, scented putty.
- Food types: Crunchy, chewy, spicy, sour, sweet, mint (be careful to consider any known allergies and dietary preferences or requirements).

Starter questions

(Starter questions for each session can be discussed either as a group as a whole or in pairs around the room.)

How does what you eat change depending on how you are feeling?

What foods do you crave when feeling stressed?

Introduction

We are looking at these two senses together due to the strong connection between them. When you pick up on a smell coming from a kitchen or a restaurant you may automatically either find it appealing and may even begin to recall the taste of that food and start to feel hungry, or be put off and move away or decide not to go into a place because of the smell. Smell is part of our natural warning system and helps us to consider if a food is safe to eat or if it has gone past its best.

Both of these senses can have a strong impact on us and help us to become more regulated or more alert. Our sense of smell has the most direct pathway to our brain and has a strong connection to our memory and emotions, and so these can be particularly effective in helping us to alter how we feel. The direct connection also leads to a quick grounding effect that can help us to feel more present. However, due to this, smells can also be triggering and caution may be needed when trialling different scents for this reason. Therefore you should not feel compelled to try anything you do not wish to.

Many of us naturally use both of these senses to self-soothe or to help us feel more awake without necessarily being aware of it. Think about how you might choose to eat chocolate when feeling stressed or to drink a fizzy drink when you want to feel energized. In this session we will trial different taste strategies and consider how we can more consciously use them to help us to go about our day and do what we need to do.

As group members trial the different items, encourage them to consider the effect each has on their arousal level and how it could be helpful. For example, could they use a certain shower gel in the morning to help them feel more awake? Or a scented room spray at night to help them to unwind?

End-of-session reflection: Ask each group member to identify one strategy they will trial using over the next week. What item have they chosen and when do they think it will be useful? Ask them to make a note of this so it can be reviewed next week.

Thank group members for their attendance and participation and inform them of the focus of the next session/agree with the group which sense they would like to focus on next.

Visual strategies
Items to bring to the session

- Pictures of different places to spark discussion: Group leaders should come prepared with a place they find visually overwhelming and one they find helpful because of the visual qualities.

- Different forms of lighting if possible – fibre optic, night light, star projector, lava lamp.
- Mandela pictures or colouring books and colouring pencils or pens.
- Examples or pictures of other activity items that could provide helpful visual input, such as cross stitch, diamond art, cooking/baking books.

Starter questions

Think about the different environments and spaces you go to – where is a place that you find calming because of what you see?

Where is a place where you find the view energizing?

Introduction

Visual input can have a big impact on us day to day as so much of what we encounter is outside of our control, but we are also very dependent on visual input. Think of how you find your way to somewhere, how you know if someone is smiling or frowning at you, and many, many more situations. We tend to choose what we wear at least partially on how it looks and what colour it is, and how that makes us feel. As with the other senses, we can learn to use visual input consciously in order to help us feel more regulated.

Participants may have a photo on their phone they wish to share of a place they find calming or energizing.

As different images are shared, encourage reflection from other group members on their response to those images/places.

Discuss different places on the ward or local to the area and how people find these. Are there any that most people find difficult or helpful? Reflect on the different reactions of group members as it is likely that different people will have a different response to the same environment. While one person may become overwhelmed by the bright lights in a fairground another person might find them energizing. Encourage group members to be as specific as possible – what features of those places make a difference? For example, is it the lighting, the number of different signs, the colours or something else?

Are there any ways in which they can manage their response to those factors or alter them? For example, would accessing a certain place at a different time alter the level of visual stimuli?

Spend time trialling some different visual items within the session that participants could use to help with certain areas, such as varying the lighting in their room.

★

End-of-session reflection: Ask each group member to identify one strategy they will trial using over the next week. What have they chosen and when do they think it will be useful? Ask them to make a note of this so it can be reviewed at the next session.

Thank group members for their attendance and participation and inform them of the focus of the next session/agree with the group which sense they would like to focus on next.

Auditory strategies
Items to bring to the session

- White noise machine/app on phone.
- A Bluetooth speaker to play music so different group members can play their choices on their phone if they wish.
- Ear defenders/headphones.
- It is helpful if you have a variety of music available to spark discussion in case group members don't bring their own or don't wish to share about their personal music.

Starter questions
What is your favourite song and why?

Is it the words/the beat/the tune you like?

Introduction
As with visual input, auditory input or noise is around us all the time and is very important in our day-to-day lives for us to interact with other people, to listen to instructions and to listen to music. Discuss how when in environments that aren't your own, or in a shared environment, it often becomes much more problematic as we then have reduced control and sounds can become much more unexpected.

Bring samples of different everyday noises to help provoke discussion and reflection – for example sea sounds, traffic noises, bird sounds. The idea of this session is to provoke discussion on the general impact auditory input has on us within our environments.

What are some ways to manage problematic sounds within the environments we need to or want to access? Acknowledge that it is not always possible to change the level of auditory stimulation within an environment – but are there ways we can manage this? Examples may include using ear defenders or ear plugs, listening to our own music on headphones, or using white noise.

This may be a good point to introduce group members to white noise. White noise is a constant, unvarying noise which can help divert our attention towards it away from other, more problematic noises. Examples include the background noise of a fan or a hoover – consider the effect this can have on infants in soothing them to sleep. White noise can have a similar calming effect on us as adults, and may be useful when we can't change the auditory features or levels in an environment, but can also be helpful for those who find complete silence difficult when trying to sleep.

Spend some time trialling a few sounds on a white noise app or machine. It would be helpful to identify potential apps before the session that group members may want to download if they find white noise helpful or wish to trial it further.

In the next part of the session we will have a think about music in particular, and how this can be helpful or unhelpful in altering our arousal levels. Reflect on some of the different times when group members like listening to music, such as on the way to work, when going for a walk or run, or when cleaning. Are there differences between the preferences within the group?

We can use music in helpful or unhelpful ways to alter our mood. Examples may be listening to energizing music to help us complete a task, or listening to certain music to intentionally indulge a mood. Discuss that the impact different types of music can have on us tends to be very individual, and we are all likely to use it in slightly different ways; we need to reflect on our own response to be able to better use it to help us to feel regulated. For example, for one person or at certain times, listening to a sad song when upset may be cathartic and help us to gain a sense of release, but at other times it could be triggering and lead to us dwelling on unhelpful thoughts and feelings. All group members are likely to already have music that they use in different ways, but the aim of this session is to start to use it more consciously to help us regulate our arousal levels.

Activity

Ask each group member to identify a song that they find helpful for when they need to be active or feel more energized, and one for when they want to unwind and relax – you could have group members create a mood board for different songs.

End-of-session reflection
Have they discovered any new types of music from other group members' choices they might try using? Will they use music any differently going forwards?

Thank group members for their attendance and participation and inform them of the focus of the next session/agree with the group which sense they would like to focus on next.

Touch strategies
Items to bring to the session

- A selection of fidget tools, e.g. tangle fidgets, stress balls, putties, hand exercisers.
- Everyday items people might fidget with, such as blue tack, paperclips, pens.
- A selection of different fabrics/materials.
- Vibration cushion or vibrating massage tool.
- Weighted item such as a weighted blanket, weighted shawl or weighted teddy.
- Different activity items or pictures of activities that may give tactile input, such as crochet, knitting, clay, baking items.

Starter questions
Do you ever find yourself fidgeting with items when trying to concentrate or when nervous?

What do you tend to fidget with?

Why do you think it helps?

Reflect that this is likely to be something we are automatically doing without being aware of it in order to regulate ourselves. We'll think about this more later in the session.

Introduction
Our touch receptors are literally everywhere so we are constantly getting touch input without consciously seeking it and with limited control over much of it. Think about all of the input you will be getting right now from your clothes, your hair, the chair you are sitting on, and so on.

Our touch system is highly important in a number of ways – it helps us form attachments to others (particularly important when we are young), it helps us to communicate with others, it helps us to be soothed or more regulated, and it helps us to understand our environment. Ask group members to identify a few ways in which touch is important in their day-to-day lives or the tasks that they need to or want to do.

Discuss that in terms of sensory processing there are different types of/ aspects of touch:

- Light touch: The tickly feel you get from your hair brushing your neck, a clothes label, someone brushing past you. This form of touch is naturally more alerting for most people as it triggers our safety system and helps us think if we need to respond to something or take action, for example brushing off a spider crawling on our skin.

- Pain and temperature: This is also a more alerting form of touch that tells our brain we need to react and make sure we are safe. Temperature can also be soothing and can reassure us – think of a hot water bottle perhaps.

- Deep pressure touch: This is the type of touch we gain from a firm hug, a massage or from rubbing our skin. This form of touch is generally more calming for people as it helps to dampen down those safety responses that are triggered by light touch, pain or other sensations. It may be helpful to mention briefly at this point that people can experience different reactions to deep touch due to factors such as experiences they have had which may have altered that natural response.

- Vibration: Similar to deep pressure touch, this works on a deeper pathway that tends to have a more regulating effect and can be helpful to regulate response to other sensory triggers.

Touch can be a highly triggering sense for individuals who have experienced trauma, so remind group members they do not have to try anything they are not comfortable with and to trust their natural reactions during the session.

Activity
Spend time allowing group members to trial the different items available. Ask them to reflect back to the window of tolerance as they do this and to think

about how using the items alters their level of arousal or could be used to help them do so.

End-of-session reflection
Are there particular items they found helpful? Did they notice themselves having a strong response to any items? Did they identify any activities they find helpful because of the touch input?

Thank group members for their attendance and participation and inform them of the focus of the next session/agree with the group which sense they would like to focus on next.

Movement strategies
Items to bring to the session

- Gym ball (peanut balls can be a helpful alternative where balance is an issue).
- Hand weights or ankle/wrist weights.
- Resistance bands.
- Wobble cushion.

Starter question
How do you feel when you spend all day in bed?

Introduction
The movement senses, vestibular input and proprioception, are often ones that people don't tend to naturally think about but are two of the most powerful sensations in altering our arousal levels. When we are thinking about movement we are considering two main senses: vestibular and proprioceptive input.

Vestibular input: Remind group members that this relates to our sense of gravity, our sense of balance and of whether we are moving or not. The receptors for our vestibular system are in our ears, so we receive vestibular input any time we move our head out of its natural position. There are two main types of vestibular input we think about, linear and rotational. Linear vestibular input is movements backwards and forwards or up and down, and tend to be more regulating when they are rhythmic and steady but become more alerting if faster or more irregular. Think about how we rock a baby to calm it and to help it to go to sleep. If we tend to become travel sick it is likely to be due to a sensitivity within this system.

Rotational vestibular input comes from movements such as spinning on a roundabout, spinning around at an activity such as an exercise or dance class, or going on a ride like the waltzers at a fair. Rotational input tends to be more intense and alerting, and more difficult to tolerate for some people.

Proprioceptive input: Remind group members that this relates to feedback we get from our muscles and gives us our awareness of where we are in space. This system is thought to be the most powerful in regulating our arousal levels and calming our response to other sensory inputs, as it has the most direct impact on our brain. Strategies that activate this system are therefore likely to be the most powerful when we are feeling agitated or anxious.

Discussion: Can group members think of any activities they do where they get these inputs? These could be sports, exercise or everyday activities such as cleaning the house or baking. Ask them to reflect on why they do this activity, particularly thinking about the physical aspects of the activity. How do they feel when doing the activity? Do they notice any changes in their mood after the activity?

It can be helpful to identify 'short, sharp' movement activities that can be used as and when an individual notices their arousal levels changing alongside more activity-based strategies that can be used to support overall regulation and can be planned into our week. During the next part of this session we are going to trial strategies in relation to each of these.

Activity

Ask group members to trial a range of the following movements. To help group members to feel less self-conscious you could create different stations around the room where they trial different movements, rather than everyone doing the same movement together at the same time. Stations could include:

- holding a plank
- doing a full push-up, wall push-up or chair push-up
- doing a squat
- using hand weights or wrist/ankle weights
- pushing against either side of a gym ball with someone else
- sitting and gently bouncing on a gym ball.

Before moving onto the main activity of the session, spend a bit of time reflecting as a group on the strategies different people have trialled and if any of them were helpful. Would they trial using any? When might they be helpful?

Choose a movement activity to trial during this session. You may wish to provide some potential ideas to group members the week before and ask them to decide on one that they will trial together. Options could include:

- yoga
- progressive muscle relaxation
- a high-intensity workout.

End-of-session reflection
How did they find the activity? Did they notice any changes in their arousal levels when doing the activity? Or now after having finished the activity?

Reassure group members that the same activity may not work for everyone and it can take trial and error to find the right movement activity for them personally.

Thank group members for their attendance and participation and inform them of the focus of the next session/agree with the group which sense they would like to focus on next, if there is more than one sense remaining to cover.

Interoception strategies
Starter questions
How can you tell when you are feeling nervous about something?

What does it feel like when you are hungry?

Introduction
Interoception is the sense that tells us about internal sensations and what is happening within our body. It is this sense that lets us know important things like when we need to eat, when we need to go to the toilet and how fast our heart is beating. It helps us to be able to meet a lot of our basic needs to keep us healthy.

This sense also helps us to understand how we are feeling in terms of our emotions as it lets us make sense of those internal cues like when we are nervous and our stomach is churning or we are starting to shake. These are connected rather than separate processes, as there is an automatic connection between our feelings and our bodies.

Being aware of our bodies' internal signals is highly important in self-regulation and managing our arousal levels and is likely to help us spot the early signs of our arousal levels increasing before it becomes problematic. The sooner we are able to spot increases in our arousal and implement a strategy to help us manage that, the more likely we will be able to avoid going into that zone of over-arousal where we are more likely to use unhelpful strategies or act impulsively.

Activity

There are a whole range of possible activities to support and develop interoceptive awareness in relation to breathing, mindfulness, temperature and more, and which ones you choose to use within the session is likely to vary depending on your client group and their potential needs. Two or three exercises are likely to give you enough discussion points to develop understanding. Potential exercises could include:

- Box breathing.
- Creating flexion and extension in an area of the body, such as your fingers or toes, and focusing on the difference in how it feels.
- Focusing on one body part while completing a movement, for example how your calf feels as you bend over at the waist and then straighten up.
- Completing an aspect of progressive muscle relaxation and focusing on how that body part feels when tensed and when relaxed.
- You could also choose to repeat one of the movements from the movement session, such as holding a plank.

After completing each of the movements or exercises, ask group members to reflect on and share what they noticed, such as where they felt tension, whether they became more aware of any body parts, whether they noticed other areas relax as they completed or after completing the movement.

End-of-session reflection

End the session by looking back at the window of tolerance. What do group members notice in their body when they are at the different levels? Is there a change in muscle tension, in their breathing? Do they feel less/more hungry or are they more likely not to notice the need to do certain things like eat or drink?

Overall reflection session

This could be done as the end part of one of the previous sessions on particular senses, but it is likely to be helpful to allow a bit of time between covering the last sense and this session so that group members can reflect on their learning and begin trialling strategies further. The main purpose of this session is to reflect in order to support group members in beginning to actively implement the strategies they have chosen and to continue developing them further. Therefore you may wish to provide an overall summary recap of the content of the group or simply to use the reflection questions below as a focus.

Suggested points of reflection:

- Look back at the notes they made on the different levels of the window of tolerance in Session 1, if they still have this, or to try and think back to what they noted. Is there more information they could add to this now? How has their understanding of what the different levels look like for them developed? And how has their awareness of what moves them between the levels improved?

- Were there certain senses they noticed as being more problematic for them? When are they more likely to be a problem? What ways have they identified to manage this? (Remember that their strategy for managing it may have come from a different sensory input!)

- Ask each group member to try and identify five different strategies they have developed through the group programme – from a variety of senses if possible. Ask them to spend time discussing in pairs the strategies they have found and when they have tried using them so far.

- Has anyone developed or identified any new strategies outside of the group that they could share with others?

- How are they going to make sure they implement the strategies they have identified? Do they need prompts from other people, or a prompt for themselves such as a sensory plan or sensory kit? What support do they need with this?

You may wish to support group members in developing a sensory plan as part of this session or outside of it, depending on the mix of group members and needs. A sensory support plan template is included in Appendix 2 to help with producing this.

Where possible it is likely to be helpful to have a follow-on review session after 4–6 weeks to review how group members are doing with using their strategies and to problem-solve any difficulties they are finding in using the strategies.

APPENDIX 4

Training Session PowerPoint

This PowerPoint presentation is designed to give you a starting point for a training session to be delivered to staff from any profession. You may wish to adapt it further to consider the needs of your specific client group or work setting. The PowerPoint presentation as shown here and the separate slides can be downloaded from https://digitalhub.jkp.com/redeem using the code KWSHBDS.

> # Introduction to sensory processing in mental health
> Staff training session template

NOTES

This PowerPoint is designed as an adaptable format for introducing staff to sensory processing who have little prior knowledge.

There are notes to accompany the slides that may help you consider points that it is helpful to raise or focus on as you go through the session, but you may choose to approach this in a different way.

Starter activity

What do you do to relax?

What do you do when you need to get going?

NOTES

The idea of this starter activity is to help consider that we all use sensory-based strategies already.

Be prepared to share a few of your own strategies as part of the discussion, including how and when you might use them.

Highlight that sensory strategy work is often about harnessing the benefits of those senses we respond well to in order to support our self-regulation.

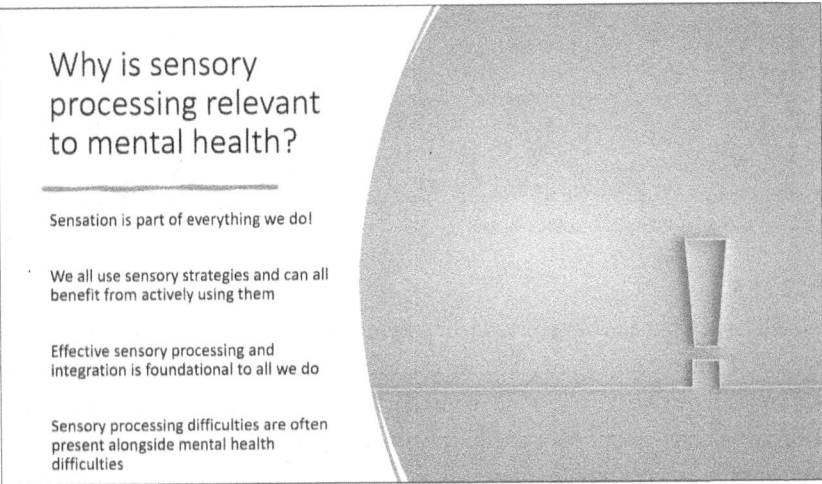

Why is sensory processing relevant to mental health?

Sensation is part of everything we do!

We all use sensory strategies and can all benefit from actively using them

Effective sensory processing and integration is foundational to all we do

Sensory processing difficulties are often present alongside mental health difficulties

NOTES

A few points to support why this is particularly relevant to consider in mental health:

- There is nothing we do that does not involve sensation.

- As considered in the starter activity, we all use sensory strategies and can all benefit from them.

- Being able to process sensory input well is central to all that we do – you may wish to highlight an example here, such as asking what senses are involved in them engaging in this training session right now.

- Sensory processing has been found to be altered alongside a range of mental health conditions.

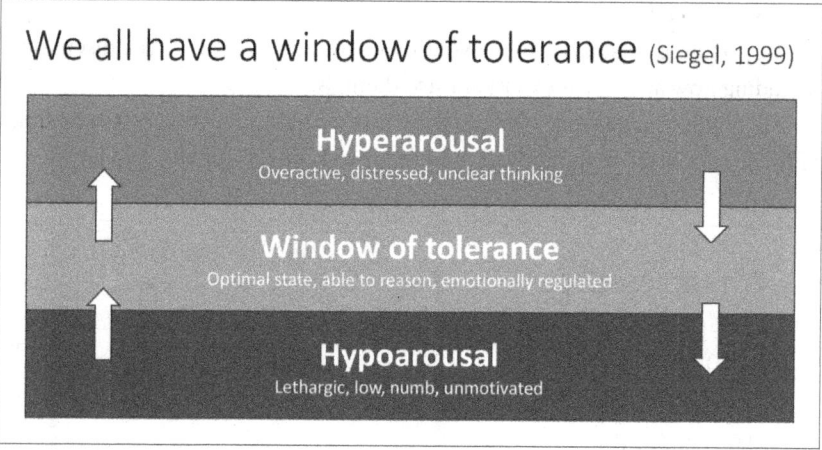

NOTES

We all have what can be referred to as a window of tolerance – that zone where we feel regulated, in a good place, we can think clearly, engage with those around us, and achieve what we need to in our day. This is that place where you can feel effective and go about your day in the way that you want, or where you can sit and engage in a training session.

We all also have zones outside of that. Hyper-arousal is the zone where we are feeling over-alert, on edge maybe, anxious or agitated. In this zone we struggle to be effective, to problem-solve, to rationalize and reason.

Below it is hypo-arousal, which is when we are feeling under-alert, and could present as quite flat, lethargic, lacking in energy and potentially in motivation.

Clients in mental health tend to be regularly moving in and out of their window of tolerance and are likely to be spending very little time in that ideal zone and far more time either hyper- or hypo-aroused.

We're going to have a think both about how sensory input can be a factor within this and also how it can help someone to better manage their movement between those zones.

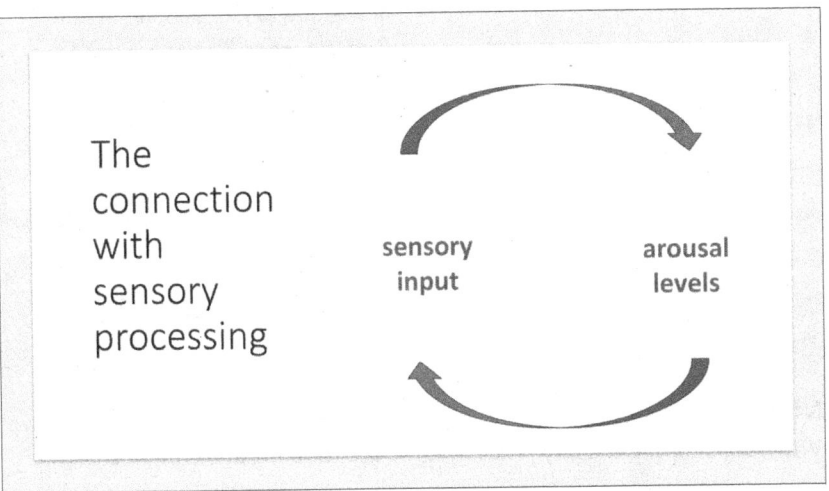

NOTES

So how does this connect to mental health? There is a cyclical relationship between sensory input and our arousal levels.

Sensory input can increase or decrease our arousal, and whether we are in a state of hyper- or hypo-arousal can alter how we respond to sensory input.

Example – think about when you are feeling stressed or over-tired. How more readily do you then respond to sensory input that you find it difficult to tolerate, such as noises of other people chattering, music you aren't in control of, or a bright light perhaps? You are going to become more easily irritated by it and your tolerance is much lower.

If you have a sensitivity or altered responsivity to sensory input in itself, this will lead to fluctuations in your arousal level also. So if you are sensitive to touch, for example, as the day progresses you may gradually become more agitated by factors such as the feel of your clothes, people brushing past you or the feel of your hair against your neck.

Now think about how it might be for someone who already has difficulties with self-regulation, like many of our clients do, and then also has difficulties with sensory responsivity. You easily end up with this vicious ongoing circle where they are constantly outside of their window of tolerance, making it very hard to do what they want to or need to do.

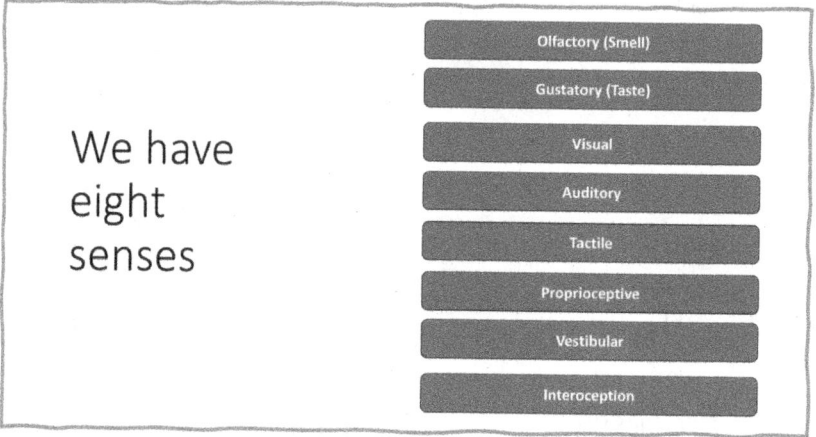

NOTES

When considering sensory processing we are thinking about eight senses:

- The five you are likely to be familiar with: olfactory (smell), gustatory (taste), vision, hearing (auditory) and tactile (touch).

- In addition to this we have two movement-based senses: proprioception, which relates to input from our muscles and joints and gives us an awareness of our bodies and position, and vestibular, which relates to our sense of balance and awareness of where we are in space and of movement.

- And lastly, interoception, which is our ability to detect internal sensations such as hunger, thirst and pain.

All of these are important in informing our understanding of ourselves and our environment, and all of these can impact on our sense of regulation. We are going to have a think about these in a bit more detail.

Taste & Olfactory

Our sense of smell and taste are closely interlinked – think how smelling food makes you start to feel hungry or can put you off your food.

Our sense of smell also has a close connection with our emotions which makes it powerful in changing how we feel.

These connections could have both a positive and negative impact on us and much of the input we receive from these senses is outside of our control.

Signs this sense may be problematic for someone: avoidance of dining halls/ cafes, strong reaction to products, narrow food choices.

NOTES

Summarize the points on the slide – particular points to highlight include how these factors are likely to be particularly problematic when someone has limited control over their environment, such as when in a hospital setting or accessing shared environments such as shops or a work place.

Auditory

Our auditory system is central to how we communicate with others but also to our sense of safety.

For an individual who spends much of their time within a hospital environment there can be many auditory stressors on a day-to-day basis that they have no control over

Signs this sense may be problematic for someone: wearing headphones much of the time, strong responses to noises such as the vacuum cleaner, people talking, keys jangling.

NOTES

Similar to the previous slide, this tends to have increased impact on our arousal when the input is outside of our control.

Discuss the potential for apparently incongruent responses – that is that someone may react strongly to noises from their environment over which they have no control but choose to play their own music, which is under their control, very loud.

Visual

Our visual system has a strong connection with other senses – particularly proprioception, vestibular and tactile

We take in a lot of visual information each day and our system can gradually become overwhelmed before we know it.

Signs this sense may be problematic for someone: wearing sunglasses, keeping the curtains closed, avoidance of bright places e.g. supermarkets

---

NOTES

It is helpful to highlight how closely this sense connects to other sensory systems, as shown on the slide.

You may wish to prompt consideration of the visual aspects of different environments and how those present in the session respond to these – helpful examples can include a supermarket, a fairground, a beach, a forest. Try to bring example pictures to support this.

Tactile (touch)

Our tactile system is our most pervasive sensory system – there are receptors everywhere and so we are constantly receiving tactile input

Tactile input is highly important in development, emotion regulation; bonding, learning, body awareness and self-soothing.

There are different types of tactile input: light touch, deep pressure touch, temperature and pain

Signs this sense may be problematic for someone: avoidance of busy areas, difficulties with self-care, inappropriate touching, layering of clothing/wearing the same clothes all the time, fussy eater.

NOTES

Discuss that our touch system can be very soothing but also very triggering, and this varies from person to person.

Highlight the strong connection this system has to our arousal levels and to forming a sense of connection with others – consider examples of how often we use our touch system when interacting, for example handshakes, a touch on the shoulder, a hug.

Draw attention to how problematic and dysregulating it is likely to be if we aren't able to process touch well.

Proprioception

Proprioception gives you your awareness of where your body is in space – it is how you know where your hand is without looking!

The receptors are in our muscles and joints and are activated by movement against resistance or heavy muscle work.

* Proprioception is highly important in regulation* and the quickest way to "ground" someone

Signs this sense may be problematic for someone: fidgety, lots of movement, physical aggression, seeking of restraint situations, low tone, poor postural control

---

NOTES

Highlight the importance of proprioception in body awareness. It may be helpful to engage those in the session in an exercise to consider the importance of this, such as completing an activity with their eyes closed and observing how much more reliant they become on feedback from their bodies.

Advise how powerful this sensation is in grounding but that it can often be forgotten in the moment. Think about how when someone is in a high state of arousal they may display behaviours that suggest they are seeking feedback from their muscles, such as physical aggression towards themselves or others, or damaging property. Can those present relate to that need to move and gain feedback from their bodies when stressed?

Vestibular

Vestibular input enables gravitational security and awareness of where we are in space

The receptors for this system are in our inner ears and are activated by movements that move the head out of midline, either linear or horizontal

Linear vestibular input tends to have a soothing effect – this is the reason we rock babies to calm them

Signs this sense may be problematic for someone: fear response when head out of midline, postural differences, rocking, pacing, risk taking behaviours, difficulty with stairs and uneven surfaces.

NOTES

Highlight the importance of vestibular input in awareness of our position in space – you could ask those present to complete an exercise where they attempt to maintain their balance with their eyes closed, such as standing on one leg.

Discuss how vestibular input can be highly soothing – the reason we rock babies.

But also discuss that it can also be very dysregulating when someone does not process it well – think about how easily this system could be stimulated due to how much we move in a day.

Interoception

Interoception is our awareness of what is going on in our body, such as hunger, thirst, pain, our heart beating.

It allows us to make sense of internal sensations and to understand our emotions - think how you know when you are anxious

Signs this sense may be problematic for someone: incontinence difficulties, missing meals/ eating too much, rapidly fluctuating emotions.

NOTES

Highlight that interoception provides awareness of both physical sensations and emotional responses, for example your stomach churning when anxious.

An individual who has difficulties with interoception is likely to struggle to interpret how they feel but also to understand the emotions of those around them.

Discussion

Out of these different senses are there any you think are particularly problematic for the people we work with?

Which of these factors are related to:
- The person themselves
- Their environment

NOTES

Points to reflect on:

- How do they see difficulties with those senses in the people they work with?
- How much of this relates to factors outside of their control?

So why do we need to understand this all better?

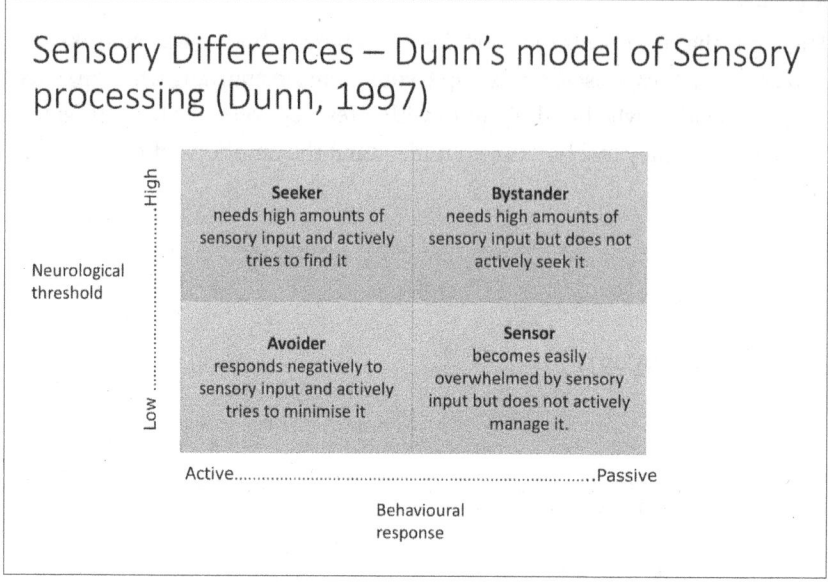

NOTES

Introduce Dunn's model as a way to understand different sensory responses.

The neurological threshold relates to our tolerance levels for sensory input. The behavioural response relates to how we manage this.

Dunn suggests four different categories of response, and how we respond will be different for each of us and depend on the sensory input, but could also vary depending on the situation. Refer to the information on the slide for what each of the categories suggests about both threshold and response. It is likely to be helpful to give examples for each; for example:

- Seeker – touches people when talking, always on the move.

- Bystander – able to focus even with a lot of noise, likely to forget things as they don't notice sensory cues as readily.

- Avoider – may leave a room if it is noisy, only eats similar foods.

- Sensor – easily distracted by noise around them, becomes overwhelmed in busy environments.

> # Discussion
>
> Which category do you think applies to you?
>
> Is this the same for all senses?

NOTES

You may want to ask participants to complete a questionnaire such as the Sensory Patterns Questionnaire in Dunn's *Living Sensationally* (Dunn, 2009) to help reflect on their own responses.

> # What approaches might be used?
>
> - Sensory support plans (sometimes called sensory diet plans)
> - Environmental adaptations
> - Timetabling or recommendation of activities
> - Education for the person or those around them
> - Further assessment of sensory needs and their impact

NOTES

On the slide are some examples of potential sensory interventions – discuss what each might involve.

- Sensory support plans – ideas of strategies the person finds helpful and when.

- Environmental adaptations – for example, changing the lighting, choosing to shop at quieter periods.

- Timetabling/activity recommendations for their sensory benefits, for example using weights in the gym for proprioceptive input.

- Education – to help the person themselves better understand their sensory responses, or for those around them so they can support the person.

- Further assessment – discuss when this might occur, for example a significant impact noted on functioning or potential connections to motor skill difficulties.

What you can do

Monitor the impact of sensory factors e.g. environmental triggers, heightened responses

Consider your impact on their sensory environment e.g. tone of voice, touch, eye contact

Support development of self-understanding

Support use of identified sensory strategies

NOTES

Highlight some ways in which they can support an individual's sensory needs:

- Considering the impact of different environments.
- Thinking about the way in which their communication with that person could be a factor and adjusting this as needed.
- Reflecting back to the person when they notice the impact of sensory factors to support increased understanding.
- Reminders to use identified strategies to help manage their arousal levels.

Points to remember

- We all have our own sensory patterns and responses
- The way in which we respond may vary for different senses and at different times

> "Sensory processing patterns are reflections of who we are: these patterns are not a pathology that needs fixing... sensory processing knowledge can narrow this gap and reduce interference, thereby affording a satisfying life."

Dunn, 2001

NOTES

Summary points for the session:

- We all have our own sensory responses that are a unique part of who we are.
- These responses may vary according to the particular sense or the situation.
- Considering sensory needs is relevant to everyone – it is not about pathologizing but about enabling someone to live their life the way they want to.

References

Dunn, W. (1997) The Impact of Sensory Processing Abilities on the Daily Lives of Young Children and Their Families: A Conceptual Model, *Infants & Young Children,* 9(4), pp. 23-35.

Dunn, W. (2001) The sensations of everyday life: empirical, theoretical and pragmatic considerations, 2001 Eleanor Clarke Slagle lecture. *American Journal of Occupational Therapy,* 55, 608-620.

Dunn, W. (2009) *Living Sensationally.* Jessica Kingsley.

Siegel (1999) *The developing mind: toward a neurobiology of interpersonal experience.* Guildford press.

References

Acevedo, B. P., Santander, T., Marhenke, R., Aron, A., & Aron, E. (2021). Sensory processing sensitivity predicts individual differences in resting-state functional connectivity associated with depth of processing. *Neuropsychobiology*, 80(2), 185–200. https://doi.org/10.1159/000513527

Alhaj, H. A., & Trist, A. (2023). The effects of sensory modulation on patient's distress and use of restrictive interventions in adult inpatient psychiatric settings: A critical review. *Advances in Biomedical and Health Sciences*, 2(3), 105–111. https://doi.org/10.4103/abhs.abhs_52_22

Ali, T., Sisay, M., Tariku, M., Mekuria, A. N., & Desalew, A. (2021). Antipsychotic-induced extrapyramidal side effects: A systematic review and meta-analysis of observational studies. *PLoS ONE*, 16(9), e0257129. https://doi.org/10.1371/journal.pone.0257129

Allee-Herndon, K. A., Dillman Taylor, D., & Roberts, S. K. (2019). Putting play in its place: Presenting a continuum to decrease mental health referrals and increase purposeful play in classrooms. *International Journal of Play*, 8(2), 186–203. https://doi.org/10.1080/21594937.2019.1643993

Alves, J., Petrosyan, A., & Magalhães, R. (2014). Olfactory dysfunction in dementia. *World Journal of Clinical Cases*, 2(11), 661–667. https://doi.org/10.12998/wjcc.v2.i11.661

American Psychiatric Association (2023, February). What are eating disorders? www.psychiatry.org/patients-families/eating-disorders/what-are-eating-disorders

American Psychiatric Association (2013). *Diagnostic and Statistical Manual of Mental Disorders* (5th ed.). American Psychiatric Publishing.

Anticevic, A., Haut, K., Murray, J. D., Repovs, G., et al. (2015). Association of thalamic dysconnectivity and conversion to psychosis in youth and young adults at elevated clinical risk. *JAMA Psychiatry*, 72(9), 882–891. https://doi.org/10.1001/jamapsychiatry.2015.0566

Asher, A. V., Parham, L. D., & Knox, S. (2008). Interrater reliability of sensory integration and praxis tests (SIPT) interpretation. *American Journal of Occupational Therapy*, 62(3), 308–319. https://doi.org/10.5014/ajot.62.3.308

Australian Health Ministers' Advisory Council (2013). *A National Framework for Recovery-Oriented Mental Health Services: Policy and Theory*. www.health.gov.au/sites/default/files/documents/2021/04/a-national-framework-for-recovery-oriented-mental-health-services-policy-and-theory.pdf

Ayres, A. J. (2005). *Sensory Integration and the Child* (25th anniversary ed.). Western Psychological Services.

Ayres, A. J. (2004). *The Sensory Integration and Praxis Tests Manual* (updated ed.). Western Psychological Services.

Ayres, A. J. (1989). *Sensory Integration and Praxis Tests*. Western Psychological Services.

Ayres, A. J. (1979). *Sensory Integration and the Child*. Western Psychological Services.

Ayres, A. J. (1972). *Sensory Integration and Learning Disorders*. Western Psychological Services.

Azuela, G., Sutton, D., & van Kessel, K. (2023). Sensory modulation implementation strategies within inpatient mental health services: An organisational case study. *Mental Health Review Journal*, 28(3), 242–256. https://doi.org/10.1108/MHRJ-06-2022-0035

Back, S. N., & Bertsch, K. (2020). Interoceptive processing in borderline personality pathology: A review on neurophysiological mechanisms. *Current Behavioural Neuroscience Reports*, 7, 232–238. https://doi.org/10.1007/s40473-020-00217-2

Bailliard, A. L. (2015). Habits of the sensory system and mental health: Understanding sensory dissonance. *American Journal of Occupational Therapy*, 69(4), 6904250020p1–6904250020p8. https://doi.org/10.5014/ajot.2015.014977

Bailliard, A., Lee, B., & Bennett, J. (2023). Polysensoriality and aesthetics: The lived sensory experiences of adults with mental illness. *Canadian Journal of Occupational Therapy*, 90(1), 103–113. https://doi.org/10.1177/00084174221145811

Bailliard, A. L., & Whigham, S. C. (2017). Linking neuroscience, function, and intervention: A scoping review of sensory processing and mental illness. *American Journal of Occupational Therapy*, 71(5), 7105100040p1–7105100040p18. https://doi.org/10.5014/ajot.2017.024497

Balaji, G. K., John, P., & Kandasamy, G. (2021). A single-center, single blinded, randomized controlled trial protocol of therapeutic listening programme versus traditional music therapy on depression and quality of life in institutionalized adolescents. *Medico-Legal Update*, 21(2). https://10.37506/mlu.v21i2.2657

Barel, E., Abu-Shkara, R., Colodner, R., Masalha, R., et al. (2018). Gonadal hormones modulate the HPA-axis and the SNS in response to psychosocial stress. *Journal of Neuroscience Research*, 96(8), 1388–1397. https://doi.org/10.1002/jnr.24259

Barker, M. S., Burke, L. J., Easterbrooks-Dick, O. K., Kane, A. W., Savrann, J. N., & May-Benson, T. A. (2015, April). *Concurrent Validity of the Adult/Adolescent Sensory History* [Poster presentation]. American Occupational Therapy Association annual conference 2015, Nashville, TN.

Baron, K., Kielhofner, G., Iyenger, A., Goldhammer, V., & Wolenski, J. (2006). *Occupational Self-assessment (OSA)* (Version 2.2). MOHO Clearinghouse.

Bear, M., Connors, B., & Paradiso, M. A. (2020). *Neuroscience: Exploring the Brain, Enhanced Edition* (4th ed.). Jones & Bartlett Learning, LLC.

Behrman, S., Chouliaras, L., & Ebmeier, K. P. (2014). Considering the senses in the diagnosis and management of dementia. *Maturitas*, 77(4), 305–310. https://doi.org/10.1016/j.maturitas.2014.01.003

Bell, K., Coulthard, H., & Wildbur, D. (2017). Self-disgust within eating disordered groups: Associations with anxiety, disgust sensitivity and sensory processing. *European Eating Disorders Review*, 25(5), 373–380. https://doi.org/10.1002/erv.2529

Bhreathnach, E. (2018, June). *Sensory Information, Sensory Integration and Strategic Functioning* [Paper presentation]. The International Association for the Study of Attachment 10th Anniversary International Conference, Florence.

Bhreathnach, E. (2009). *Trauma, Sensory Processing & Attachment: Sensory-Attachment Intervention* [Paper presentation]. Family Futures Conference, London.

Bhreathnach, E. (2008). *Parent–Child Engagement, A Co-Regulation Process* [Paper presentation]. The National Conference for Occupational Therapists in Child and Adolescent Mental Health, Northampton, UK.

Bilek, E., Itz, M. L., Stoßel, G., Ma, R., et al. (2019). Deficient amygdala habituation to threatening stimuli in borderline personality disorder relates to adverse childhood experiences. *Biological Psychiatry*, 86(12), 930–938. https://doi.org/10.1016/j.biopsych.2019.06.008

Birba, A., Santamaría-García, H., Prado, P., Cruzat, J., et al. (2022). Allostatic-interoceptive overload in frontotemporal dementia. *Biological Psychiatry*, 92(1), 54–67. https://doi.org/10.1016/j.biopsych.2022.02.955

Blanche, E. I. (2010). *Observations Based on Sensory Integration Theory* (2nd ed.). Pediatric Therapy Network.

Blanche, E. I., Parham, D., Chang, M., & Mallinson, T. (2014). Development of an adult sensory processing scale (ASPS). *American Journal of Occupational Therapy*, 68(5), 531–538. https://doi.org/10.5014/ajot.2014.012484

Blanche, E. I., Reinoso, G., & Kiefer, D. B. (2021). *Structured Observations of Sensory Integration – Motor (SOSI-M)*. Academic Therapy Publications.

Blanche, E. I., Reinoso, G., & Kiefer, D. B. (2020). Using Clinical Observations Within the Evaluation Process. In A. C. Bundy & S. J. Lane (eds), *Sensory Integration: Theory and Practice* (3rd ed.) (pp. 222–242). F. A. Davis.

Blanche, E. I., & Schaaf, R. C. (2001). Proprioception: A Cornerstone of Sensory Integrative Intervention. In S. Smith Roley, E. I. Blanche & R. C. Schaaf (eds), *Sensory Integration with Diverse Populations* (pp. 109–124). Pro-ed.

Borghammer, P., Horsager, J., Andersen, K., Van Den Berge, N., et al. (2021). Neuropathological evidence of body-first vs. brain-first Lewy body disease. *Neurobiology of Disease*, 161, 105557. https://doi.org/10.1016/j.nbd.2021.105557

Bosch, J. (1995). *The Reliability and Validity of the COPM* [Master's thesis]. McMaster University. Hamilton, Ontario.

Brand-Gothelf, A., Parush, S., Eitan, Y., Admoni, S., Gur, E., & Stein, D. (2016). Sensory modulation disorder symptoms in anorexia nervosa and bulimia nervosa: A pilot study. *International Journal of Eating Disorders*, 49(1), 59–68. https://doi.org/10.1002/eat.22460

Breckenridge, J., & Jones, D. (2015). Evaluation in everyday occupational therapy practice: Should we be thinking about treatment fidelity? *British Journal of Occupational Therapy*, 78(5), 331-333. https://doi.org/10.1177/0308022614562583

Brockmeyer, T., Friederich, H. C., & Schmidt, U. (2018). Advances in the treatment of anorexia nervosa: A review of established and emerging interventions. *Psychological Medicine*, 48(8), 1228-1256. https://doi.org/10.1017/S0033291717002604

Brown, A., Tse, T., & Fortune, T. (2018). Defining sensory modulation: A review of the concept and a contemporary definition for application by occupational therapists. *Scandinavian Journal of Occupational Therapy*, 26(7), 515-523. https://doi.org/10.1080/11038128.2018.1509370

Brown, C. (2020). Adolescent/Adult Sensory Profile. In B. J. Hemphill & C. K. Urish (eds), *Assessments in Occupational Therapy Mental Health: An Integrative Approach* (4th ed.) (pp. 468-479). Taylor & Francis.

Brown, C., Cromwell, R. L., Filion, D., Dunn, W., & Tollefson, N. (2002). Sensory processing in schizophrenia: Missing and avoiding information. *Schizophrenia Research*, 55(1-2), 187-195. https://doi.org/10.1016/s0920-9964(01)00255-9

Brown, C., & Dunn, W. (2023). Development of a participation focused measure of interoception for adults. *OTJR: Occupational Therapy Journal of Research*, 43(2), 264-270. https://doi.org/10.1177/15394492221112651

Brown, C. E., & Dunn, W. (2002). *Adolescent/Adult Sensory Profile*. Pearson.

Brown, J. (2011). Talking about life after early psychosis: The impact on occupational performance. *Canadian Journal of Occupational Therapy*, 78, 156-163. https://doi.org/10.2182/cjot.2011.78.3.3

Brown, S., Shankar, R., & Smith, K. (2009). Borderline personality disorder and sensory processing impairment. *Progress in Neurology and Psychiatry*, 13, 10-16. https://doi.org/10.1002/pnp.127

Brown, T., Almiento, L., Yu, M., & Bhopti, A. (2023). The Sensory Processing Measure - Second Edition: A Critical Review and Appraisal. *Occupational Therapy in Health Care*, 38(3), 842-875. https://doi.org/10.1080/07380577.2023.2280216

Brown, T. A., Berner, L. A., Jones, M. D., Reilly, E. E., et al. (2017). Psychometric evaluation and norms for the Multidimensional Assessment of Interoceptive Awareness (MAIA) in a clinical eating disorders sample. *European Eating Disorders Review*, 25(5), 411-416. https://doi.org/10.1002/erv.2532

Bugajska, K., & Brooks, R. (2021). Evaluating the use of the Model of Human Occupation Screening Tool in mental health services. *British Journal of Occupational Therapy*, 84(9), 591-600. https://doi.org/10.1177/0308022620956580

Bundy, A. C., & Lane, S. J. (2020). Sensory Integration: A. Jean Ayres' Theory Revisited. In A. C. Bundy & S. J. Lane (eds), *Sensory Integration: Theory and Practice* (3rd ed.) (pp. 2-20). F. A. Davis.

Bundy, A. C., & Szklut, S. (2020). The Science of Intervention: Creating Direct Intervention from Theory. In A. C. Bundy & S. J. Lane (eds), *Sensory Integration: Theory and Practice* (3rd ed.) (pp. 300-335). F. A. Davis.

Buysse, D. J., Reynolds III, C. F., Monk, T. H., Berman, S. R., & Kupfer, D. J. (1989). The Pittsburgh Sleep Quality Index: A new instrument for psychiatric practice and research. *Psychiatry Research*, 28(2), 193-213. https://doi.org/10.1016/0165-1781(89)90047-4

Carter, O., Bennett, D., Nash, T., Arnold, S., et al. (2017). Sensory integration deficits support a dimensional view of psychosis and are not limited to schizophrenia. *Translational Psychiatry*, 7(5), e1118-e1118. https://doi.org/10.1038/tp.2017.69

Cerejeira, J., Lagarto, L., & Mukaetova-Ladinska, E. B. (2012). Behavioral and psychological symptoms of dementia. *Frontiers in Neurology*, 3(73). https://doi.org/10.3389/fneur.2012.00073

Cermak, S. (1992). Sensory integration with the adult: Application and misapplication. *Israel Journal of Occupational Therapy*, 1(3), E57-E74.

Cermak, S., & May-Benson, T. (2020). Praxis and Dyspraxia. In A. C. Bundy & S. J. Lane (eds), *Sensory Integration: Theory and Practice* (3rd ed.) (pp. 115-150). F. A. Davis.

Chalmers, A., Harrison, S., Mollison, K., Molloy, V., & Gray, K. (2012). Establishing sensory-based approaches in mental health inpatient care: A multidisciplinary approach. *Australasian Psychiatry*, 20(1), 35-39. https://doi.org/10.1177/1039856211430146

Champagne, T. (2018). *Sensory Modulation in Dementia Care*. Jessica Kingsley Publishers.

Champagne, T. (2011). The influence of posttraumatic stress disorder, depression, and sensory processing patterns on occupational engagement: A case study. *Work*, 38(1), 67-75. https://doi.org/10.3233/WOR-2011-1105

Champagne, T., & Koomar, J. (2012). Evaluating sensory processing in mental health. *OT Practice*, 17(5), 1-8.

Champagne, T., Koomar, J., & Olson, L. (2010). Sensory processing evaluation and intervention in mental health. *OT Practice*, 15(5), CE-1-CE-8.

Champagne, T., & Pfeiffer, B. (2020). Sensory Integration Approaches with Adults with Mental Health Disorders. In A. C. Bundy & S. J. Lane (eds), *Sensory Integration Theory and Practice* (3rd ed.) (pp. 513–530). F. A. Davis.

Cheng, C. H., Chan, P. Y. S., Liu, C. Y., & Hsu, S. C. (2016). Auditory sensory gating in patients with bipolar disorders: A meta-analysis. *Journal of Affective Disorders*, 203, 199–203. https://doi.org/10.1016/j.jad.2016.06.010

Cherian, K., Schatzberg, A. F., & Keller, J. (2019). HPA axis in psychotic major depression and schizophrenia spectrum disorders: Cortisol, clinical symptomatology, and cognition. *Schizophrenia Research*, 213, 72–79. https://doi.org/10.1016/j.schres.2019.07.003

Chung, J. C. C. (2006). Measuring sensory processing patterns of older Chinese people: Psychometric validation of the adult sensory profile. *Aging and Mental Health*, 10(6), 648–655. https://doi.org/10.1080/13607860600648080

Clifford, C., Paulk, E., Lin, Q., Cadwallader, J., Lubbers, K., & Frazier, L. D. (2024). Relationships among adult playfulness, stress, and coping during the COVID-19 pandemic. *Current Psychology*, 43(9), 8403–8412. https://doi.org/10.1007/s12144-022-02870-0

Cobbaert, L., Hay, P., Mitchell, P. B., Roza, S. J., & Perkes, I. (2024). Sensory processing across eating disorders: A systematic review and meta-analysis of self-report inventories. *International Journal of Eating Disorders*, 54, 1456–1488. https://doi.org/10.1002/eat.24184

Cobbaert, L., & Rose, A. (2023). *Eating Disorders and Neurodivergence: A Stepped Care Approach*. https://nedc.com.au/assets/NEDC-Publications/Eating-Disorders-and-Neurodivergence-A-Stepped-Care-Approach.pdf

Colle, L., Hilviu, D., Rossi, R., Garbarini, F., & Fossataro, C. (2020). Self-harming and sense of agency in patients with borderline personality disorder. *Frontiers in Psychiatry*, 11, 449–449. https://doi.org/10.3389/fpsyt.2020.00449

Collier, L., McPherson, K., Ellis-Hill, C., Staal, J., & Bucks, R. (2010). Multisensory stimulation to improve functional performance in moderate to severe dementia – interim results. *American Journal of Alzheimer's Disease and Other Dementias*, 25(8), 698–703. https://doi.org/10.1177/1533317510387582

Cooper, J., Parkinson, S., de las Heras de Pablo, C. G., Shute, R., Melton, J., & Forsyth, K. (2018). *A User's Manual for the Model of Human Occupation Exploratory Level Outcome Ratings (MOHO-ExpLOR)*. NHS Lothian & Queen Margaret University.

Correia, C., Lopez, K., Wroblewski, M., Huisingh-Scheetz, M., & Kern, D. (2016). Global sensory impairment in older adults in the United States. *Journal of the American Geriatrics Society*, 64(2), 306–313. https://doi.org/10.1111/jgs.13955

Costantini, M., Salone, A., Martinotti, G., Fiori, F., et al. (2020). Body representations and basic symptoms in schizophrenia. *Schizophrenia Research*, 222, 267–273. https://doi.org/10.1016/j.schres.2020.05.038

Cox, A., Heron, T., & Frederico, M. (2024). Sensory processing assessment and feedback in the treatment of complex developmental trauma. *Journal of Child and Adolescent Trauma*, 17, 677–690. https://doi.org/10.1007/s40653-023-00607-0

Cozolino, L. (2017). *The Neuroscience of Psychotherapy*. Norton.

Crail-Melendez, D., Atriano-Mendieta, C., Carrillo-Meza, R., & Ramirez-Bermudez, J. (2013). Schizophrenia-like psychosis associated with right lacunar thalamic infarct. *Neurocase*, 19(1), 22–26. https://doi.org/10.1080/13554794.2011.654211

Craswell, G., Dieleman, C., & Ghanouni, P. (2021). An integrative review of sensory approaches in adult inpatient mental health: Implications for occupational therapy in prison-based mental health services. *Occupational Therapy in Mental Health*, 37(2), 130–157. https://doi.org/10.1080/0164212X.2020.1853654

Crittenden, P., & Landini, A. (2011). *Assessing Adult Attachment: A Dynamic-Maturational Approach to Discourse Analysis*. Norton.

Cromwell, R. L. (1993). Searching for the origins of schizophrenia. *Psychological Science*, 4(5), 276–279. https://doi.org/10.1111/j.1467-9280.1993.tb00563.x

Crowe, J. (2014). Professional reasoning and occupational therapist's use of a multi-sensory environment for clients with dementia. *Physical and Occupational Therapy in Geriatrics*, 32(3), 198–209. https://doi.org/10.3109/02703181.2014.927947

Cusic, E., Hoppe, M., Sultenfuss, M., Jacobs, K., Holler, H., & Obembe, A. (2022). Multisensory environments for outcomes of occupational engagement in dementia: A systematic review. *Physical and Occupational Therapy in Geriatrics*, 40(3), 275–294. https://doi.org/10.1080/02703181.2022.2028954

Dark, E., & Carter, S. (2020). Shifting identities: Exploring occupational identity for those in recovery from an eating disorder. *Qualitative Research Journal*, 20(1), 127–139. https://doi.org/10.1108/QRJ-07-2019-0054

de Beurs, E., Carlier, I., & van Hemert, A. (2022). Psychopathology and health-related quality of life as patient-reported treatment outcomes: Evaluation of concordance between the Brief Symptom Inventory (BSI) and the Short Form-36 (SF-36) in psychiatric outpatients. *Quality of Life Research*, 31, 1461–1471. https://doi.org/10.1007/s11136-021-03019-5

De Lecea, L., Carter, M. E., & Adamantidis, A. (2012). Shining a light on wakefulness and arousal. *Biological Psychiatry*, 71(12), 1046–1052. https://doi.org/10.1016/j.biopsych.2012.01.032

Dean, E. E., Little, L., Tomchek, T., & Dunn, W. (2018). Sensory processing in the general population: Adaptability, resiliency, and challenging behaviour. *American Journal of Occupational Therapy*, 72(1), 1–8. https://doi.org/10.5014/ajot.2018.019919

Dementia UK (2024). Types of Dementia. www.dementiauk.org/information-and-support/types-of-dementia

Dempsey, A. (2016). An Evaluation of a Brief Sensory Modulation Intervention for People Presenting With Anxiety in a Community Mental Health Service [Unpublished masters dissertation]. Auckland University of Technology. https://openrepository.aut.ac.nz/server/api/core/bitstreams/f20cb78f-9554-42e8-9549-4655f649a43d/content

Dimitriou, T., Papatriantafyllou, J., Konsta, A., Kazis, D., et al. (2022). Non-pharmacological interventions for wandering/aberrant motor behaviour in patients with dementia. *Brain Science*, 12, 130. https://doi.org/10.3390/brainsci12020130

Dintica, C. S., Marseglia, A., Rizzuto, D., Wang, R., et al. (2019). Impaired olfaction is associated with cognitive decline and neurodegeneration in the brain. *Neurology*, 92(7), e700–e709. https://doi.org/10.1212/WNL.0000000000006919

Dobinson, A., Cooper, M., & Quesnel, D. A. (2019). *Safe Exercise at Every Stage Guidelines (SEES)*. www.safeexerciseateverystage.com

Dorn, E., Hitch, D., & Stevenson, C. (2020). An evaluation of a sensory room within an adult mental health rehabilitation unit. *Occupational Therapy in Mental Health*, 36(2), 105–118. https://doi.org/10.1080/0164212X.2019.1666770

Doroud, N., Cappy, M., Grant, K., Scopelliti, M., McKinstry, C., & McMahon, D. (2024). Sensory rooms within mental health settings: A systematic scoping review. *Occupational Therapy in Mental Health*, 1–21. https://doi.org/10.1080/0164212X.2024.2308290

Drews, E., Fertuck, E. A., Koenig, J., Kaess, M., & Arntz, A. (2019). Hypothalamic-pituitary-adrenal axis functioning in borderline personality disorder: A meta-analysis. *Neuroscience and Biobehavioural Reviews*, 96, 316–334. https://doi.org/10.1016/j.neubiorev.2018.11.008

Duhn, L. (2010). The importance of touch in the development of attachment. *Advances in Neonatal Care*, 10(6), 294–300. https://doi.org/10.1097/ANC.0b013e3181fd2263

Duncan, E. A., & Murray, J. (2012). The barriers and facilitators to routine outcome measurement by allied health professionals in practice: A systematic review. *BMC Health Services Research*, 12(1), 1–9. https://doi.org/10.1186/1472-6963-12-96

Dunn, W. (2009). *Living Sensationally: Understanding Your Senses*. Jessica Kingsley Publishers.

Dunn, W. (2007). Supporting children to participate successfully in everyday life by using sensory processing knowledge. *Infants and Young Children*, 20(2), 84–101. https://doi.org/10.1097/01.IYC.0000264477.05076.5d

Dunn, W. (2001). The sensations of everyday life: Empirical, theoretical and pragmatic considerations. 2001 Eleanor Clarke Slagle lecture. *American Journal of Occupational Therapy*, 55, 608–620. https://doi.org/10.5014/ajot.55.6.608

Dunn, W. (1997). The impact of sensory processing abilities on the daily lives of young children and their families: A conceptual model. *Infants and Young Children*, 9(4), 23–35. https://doi.org/10.1097/00001163-199704000-00005

Dunn, W., Brown, C., Breitmeyer, A., & Salwei, A. (2022). Construct validity of the Sensory Profile Interoception Scale: Measuring sensory processing in everyday life. *Frontiers in Psychology*, 13. https://doi.org/10.3389/fpsyg.2022.872619

Elias, G. J., Giacobbe, P., Boutet, A., Germann, J., et al. (2020). Probing the circuitry of panic with deep brain stimulation: Connectomic analysis and review of the literature. *Brain Stimulation*, 13(1), 10–14. https://doi.org/10.1016/j.brs.2019.09.010

Engel-Yeger, B., Bloch, B., Gonda, X., Canepa, G., et al. (2018). Sensory profiles in unipolar and bipolar affective disorders: Possible predictors of response to antidepressant medications? A prospective follow-up study. *Journal of Affective Disorders*, 240, 237–246. https://doi.org/10.1016/j.jad.2018.07.032

Engel-Yeger, B., & Dunn, W. (2011). The relationship between sensory processing difficulties and anxiety level of healthy adults. *British Journal of Occupational Therapy*, 74(5), 210–216. https://doi.org/10.4276/030802211X13046730116

Engel-Yeger, B., Hus, S., & Rosenblum, S. (2012). Age effects on sensory-processing abilities and their impact on handwriting. *Canadian Journal of Occupational Therapy, 79*, 264-274. https://doi.org/10.2182/CJOT.2012.79.5.2

Engel-Yeger, B., Palgy-Levin, D., & Lev-Wiesel, R. (2015). Predicting fears of intimacy among individuals with post-traumatic stress symptoms by their sensory profile. *British Journal of Occupational Therapy, 78*(1), 51-57. https://doi.org/10.1177/0308022614557

Engel-Yeger, B., Palgy-Levin, D., & Lev-Wiesel, R. (2013). The sensory profile of people with post-traumatic stress symptoms. *Occupational Therapy in Mental Health, 29*(3), 266-278. https://doi.org/10.1080/0164212X.2013.819366

Engel-Yeger, B., & Shochat, T. (2012). The relationship between sensory processing patterns and sleep quality in healthy adults. *Canadian Journal of Occupational Therapy, 79*(3), 134-141. https://doi.org/10.2182/cjot.2012.79.3.2

Eshkevari, E., Rieger, E., Longo, M. R., Haggard, P., & Treasure, J. (2014). Persistent body image disturbance following recovery from eating disorders. *International Journal of Eating Disorders, 47*(4), 400-409. https://doi.org/10.1002/eat.22219

Feldman, R., Schreiber, S., Pick, C. G., & Been, E. (2020). Gait, balance and posture in major mental illnesses: Depression, anxiety and schizophrenia. *Austin Medical Sciences, 5*(1), 1-6.

Fisher, A. G. (2010). *Assessment of Motor and Process Skills. Vol. 2: User Manual* (7th ed.). Three Star Press.

Fisher, A. G. (2006). *Assessment of Motor and Process Skills. Vol. 1: Development, Standardization, and Administration Manual* (6th ed.). Three Star Press.

Fisher, A. G. (1991). Vestibular-Proprioceptive Processing and Bilateral Integration and Sequencing Deficits. In A. G. Fisher, E. A. Murray & A. C. Bundy (eds), *Sensory Integration: Theory and Practice* (pp. 71-104). F. A. Davis.

Flasbeck, V., Popkirov, S., Ebert, A., & Brüne, M. (2020). Altered interoception in patients with borderline personality disorder: A study using heartbeat-evoked potentials. *Borderline Personality Disorder and Emotion Dysregulation, 7*(1), 1-13. https://doi.org/10.1186/s40479-020-00139-1

Fletcher, P. D., Downey, L. E., Golden, H. L., Clark, C. N., et al. (2015). Pain and temperature processing in dementia: A clinical and neuroanatomical analysis. *Brain, 138*(11), 3360-3372. https://doi.org/10.1093/brain/awv276

Fraser, K., MacKenzie, D., & Versnel, J. (2017). Complex trauma in children and youth: A scoping review of sensory-based interventions. *Occupational Therapy in Mental Health, 33*(3), 199-216. https://doi.org/10.1080/0164212X.2016.1265475

French, P., Smith, J., Shiers, D., Reed, M., & Rayne, M. (2010). *Promoting Recovery in Early Psychosis: A Practice Manual*. Wiley-Blackwell.

Frick, S. M. (2020). Therapeutic Listening®. In A. C. Bundy & S. J. Lane (eds), *Sensory Integration Theory and Practice* (3rd ed.) (pp. 462-466). F. A. Davis.

Frick, S. M., & Hacker, C. (2001). *Listening With the Whole Body*. Vital Links.

Galiana-Simal, A., Muñoz-Martinez, V., & Beato-Fernandez, L. (2017). Connecting eating disorders and sensory processing disorder: A sensory eating disorder hypothesis. *Global Journal of Intellectual and Developmental Disabilities, 3*(4), 1077-1087.

Gaudio, S., Brooks, S. J., & Riva, G. (2014). Nonvisual multisensory impairment of body perception in anorexia nervosa: A systematic review of neuropsychological studies. *PloS One, 9*(10). https://doi.org/10.1371/journal.pone.0110087

Gaur, N., John, P., & Kandasamy, G. (2021). Effects of therapeutic listening on depression and physical activity in school going adolescents: A randomized controlled trial. *Turkish Journal of Physiotherapy and Rehabilitation, 32*(3), 3976-3987.

Giannopoulou, I., Georgiades, S., Stefanou, M. I., Spandidos, D. A., & Rizos, E. (2023). Links between trauma and psychosis (review). *Experimental and Therapeutic Medicine, 26*, 328. https://doi.org/10.3892/etm.2023.12085

Gibbs, G. (1988). *Learning By Doing: A Guide to Teaching and Learning Methods*. FEU.

Good, K. P., Tibbo, P., Milliken, H., Whitehorn, D., et al. (2010). An investigation of a possible relationship between olfactory identification deficits at first episode and four-year outcomes in patients with psychosis. *Schizophrenia Research, 124*(1-3), 60-65. https://doi.org/10.1016/j.schres.2010.07.010

Guitard, P., Ferland, F., & Dutil, É. (2005). Toward a better understanding of playfulness in adults. *OTJR: Occupation, Participation and Health, 25*(1), 9-22. https://doi.org/10.1177/153944920502500103

Haig, S., & Hallett, N. (2023). Use of sensory rooms in adult psychiatric inpatient settings: A systematic review and narrative synthesis. *International Journal of Mental Health Nursing, 32*(1), 54-75. https://doi.org/10.1111/inm.13065

Haigh, J., & Mighton, C. (2016). Sensory interventions to support the wellbeing of people with dementia: A critical review. *British Journal of Occupational Therapy, 79*(2), 120–126. https://doi.org/10.1177/0308022615598996

Halperin, L., & Falk-Kessler, J. (2020). Schizophrenia spectrum disorders: Linking motor and process skills, sensory patterns, and psychiatric symptoms. *Open Journal of Occupational Therapy, 8*(1), 1–13. https://doi.org/10.15453/2168-6408.1659

Harrichan, S., McKinnon, M. C., & Lanius, R. C. (2021). How processing of sensory information from the internal and external worlds shape the perception and engagement with the world in the aftermath of trauma: Implications for PTSD. *Frontiers in Neuroscience*. https://doi.org/10.3389/fnins.2021.625490

Harrison, L. A., Kats, A., Williams, M. E., & Aziz-Zadeh, L. (2019). The importance of sensory processing in mental health: A proposed addition to the research domain criteria (RDoC) and suggestions for RDoC 2.0. *Frontiers in Psychology, 10*. https://doi.org/10.3389/fpsyg.2019.00103

Hart, N., McGowan, J., Minati, L., & Critchley, H. D. (2013). Emotional regulation and bodily sensation: Interoceptive awareness is intact in borderline personality disorder. *Journal of Personality Disorders, 27*(4), 506–518. https://doi.org/101521pedi201226049

Hazelton, J. L., Fittipaldi, S., Fraile-Vazquez, M., Sourty, M., et al. (2023). Thinking versus feeling: How interoception and cognition influence emotion recognition in behavioural-variant frontotemporal dementia, Alzheimer's disease, and Parkinson's disease. *Cortex, 163*, 66–79. https://doi.org/10.1016/j.cortex.2023.02.009

Health and Safety Executive (HSE) (2019). *HSE National Clinical Programme for Early Intervention in Psychosis: Model of Care*. www.hse.ie/eng/about/who/cspd/ncps/mental-health/psychosis/resources/hse-early-intervention-in-psychosis-model-of-care-june-20191.pdf

Herbert, B. M. (2020). Interoception and its role for eating, obesity, and eating disorders. *European Journal of Health Psychology, 27*(4). https://doi.org/10.1027/2512-8442/a000062

Hocking, C. (2001). The issue is implementing occupation-based assessment. *American Journal of Occupational Therapy, 55*(4), 463–469. https://doi.org/10.5014/ajot.55.4.463

Hofmann, S. G., & Bitran, S. (2007). Sensory-processing sensitivity in social anxiety disorder: Relationship to harm avoidance and diagnostic subtypes. *Journal of Anxiety Disorders, 21*(7), 944–954. https://doi.org/10.1016/j.janxdis.2006.12.003

Holland, C. M., & May-Benson, T. (2014). Rationale for integrating attachment, trauma, and sensory integration theory. Spiral Foundation Self-Study Article. Spiral Foundation.

Holland, J., Begin, D., Orris, D., & Meyer, A. (2018). A descriptive analysis of the theory and processes of an innovative day program for young women with trauma-related symptoms. *Occupational Therapy in Mental Health, 34*(3), 228–241. https://doi.org/10.1080/0164212X.2017.1393369

Hollands, T., Sutton, D., Wright-St. Clair, V., & Hall, R. (2015). Maori mental health consumers' sensory experience of Kapa Haka and its utility to occupational therapy practice. *New Zealand Journal of Occupational Therapy, 62*(1), 3–11.

Horga, G., & Abi-Dargham, A. (2019). An integrative framework for perceptual disturbances in psychosis. *Nature Reviews Neuroscience, 20*(12), 763–778. https://doi.org/10.1038/s41583-019-0234-1

Howard, A. R. H., Lynch, A. K., Call, C. D., & Cross, D. R. (2020). Sensory processing in children with a history of maltreatment: An occupational therapy perspective. *Vulnerable Children and Youth Studies, 15*(1), 60–67. https://doi.org/10.1080/17450128.2019.1687963

Hsu, Y. T., & Nelson, D. L. (1981). Adult performance on the Southern California Kinesthesis And Tactile Perception Tests. *American Journal of Occupational Therapy, 35*(12), 788–791. https://doi.org/10.5014/ajot.35.12.788

Hughes, S. (2010). Approaches to Severe and Enduring Mental Illness. In J. Creek & L. Lougher (eds), *Occupational Therapy and Mental Health* (4th ed.) (pp. 408–602). Churchill Livingstone.

Hughes, S., Woods, B., Algar-Skaife, K., & Jones, C. H. (2023). Understanding quality of life and well-being for people living with advanced dementia. *Nursing Older People, 35*(5). http://doi.org/10.7748/nop.2019.e1129

Jagiellowicz, J., Acevedo, B. P., Tillmann, T., Aron, A., & Aron, E. N. (2024). The relationship between sensory processing sensitivity and medication sensitivity: Brief report. *Frontiers in Psychology, 14*. https://doi.org/10.3389/fpsyg.2023.1320695

Jakob, A., & Collier, L. (2017). Sensory enrichment for people living with dementia: Increasing the benefits of multisensory environments in dementia care through design. *Design for Health, 1*(1), 115–133. https://doi.org/10.1080/24735132.2017.1296274

Jakob, A., & Collier, L. (2014). *How to Make a Sensory Room for People Living With Dementia: A Guide Book*. https://assets.kingston.ac.uk/m/8239cb81e12f2cb/original/How-to-make-a-Sensory-Room-for-people-with-dementia.pdf

Javitt, D. C., & Freedman, R. (2015). Sensory processing dysfunction in the personal experience and neuronal machinery of schizophrenia. *American Journal of Psychiatry*, 172(1), 17–31. https://doi.org/10.1176/appi.ajp.2014.13121691

Jenkinson, P. M., Taylor, L., & Laws, K. R. (2018). Self-reported interoceptive deficits in eating disorders: A meta-analysis of studies using the eating disorder inventory. *Journal of Psychosomatic Research*, 110, 38–45. https://doi.org/10.1016/j.jpsychores.2018.04.005

Jonsdottir, T., & Gunnarsson, E. C. (2021). Understanding nurses' knowledge and attitudes toward pain assessment in dementia: A literature review. *Pain Management Nursing*, 22(3), 281–292. https://doi.org/10.1016/j.pmn.2020.11.002

Joseph, R. Y., Casteleijn, D., van der Linde, J., & Franzsen, D. (2021). Sensory modulation dysfunction in child victims of trauma: A scoping review. *Journal of Child and Adolescent Trauma*, 14, 455–470. https://doi.org/10.1007/s40653-020-00333-x

Joseph, R. Y., van der Linde, J., & Franzsen, D. (2022). Sensory modulation dysfunction in child victims of trauma from four residential care sites in southern Gauteng, South Africa. *South African Journal of Occupational Therapy*, 52(2). https://doi.org/10.17159/2310-3833/2022/vol52n2a6

Karaca Dinç, P., Oktay, S., & Durak Batıgün, A. (2021). Mediation role of alexithymia, sensory processing sensitivity and emotional-mental processes between childhood trauma and adult psychopathology: A self-report study. *BMC Psychiatry*, 21(1), 1–10. https://doi.org/10.1186/s12888-021-03532-4

Karssemeijer, E. G. A., Aaronson, J. A., Bossers, W. J. R., Donders, R., et al. (2019). The quest for synergy between physical exercise and cognitive stimulation via exergaming in people with dementia: A randomized control study. *Alzheimer's Research and Therapy*, 11(3). https://doi.org/10.1186/s13195-018-0454-z

Kearney, B. E., & Lanius, R. A. (2022). The brain-body disconnect: A somatic sensory basis for trauma-related disorders. *Frontiers in Neuroscience*, 16. https://doi.org/10.3389/fnins.2022.1015749

Kennedy, J. (2020). Section 4: Sensory Integration and Children With Disorders of Trauma and Attachment. In A. C. Bundy & S. J. Lane (eds), *Sensory Integration Theory and Practice* (3rd ed.) (pp. 502–507). F. A. Davis.

Keptner, K. M., Fitzgibbon, C., & O'Sullivan, J. (2021). Effectiveness of anxiety reduction interventions on test anxiety: A comparison of four techniques incorporating sensory modulation. *British Journal of Occupational Therapy*, 84(5), 289–297. https://doi.org/10.1177/0308022620935061

Khalsa, S. S., Adolphs, R., Cameron, O. G., Critchley, H. D., et al. (2018). Interoception and mental health: A roadmap. *Biological Psychiatry: Cognitive Neuroscience and Neuroimaging*, 3(6), 501–513. https://doi.org/10.1016/j.bpsc.2017.12.004

Khalsa, S. S., & Feinstein, J. S. (2019). The Somatic Error Hypothesis of Anxiety. In M. Tsakiris & H. De Preester (eds), *The Interoceptive Mind: From Homeostasis to Awareness* (pp. 144–161). Oxford University Press.

Khodabakhsh, S., & Cheong, L. S. (2017). The relationship between sensory processing patterns and depression in adults. *MOJPC: Malaysia Online Journal of Psychology and Counselling*, 3(1), 49–56.

Khodarahimi, S., Mirderikvand, F., & Amraei, K. (2021). Negative affectivity, sensory processing hypersensitivity, sleep quality and dreams: A conceptual model for generalised anxiety disorder in adults. *Current Psychology*, 1–10. https://doi.org/10.1007/s12144-021-01428-w

Khoweiled, A. A., Gaafar, Y., El Makawi, S. M., Kamel, R. M., & Ayoub, D. R. (2021). Neurological soft signs correlation with symptom severity in borderline personality disorder. *Middle East Current Psychiatry*, 28, 2. https://doi.org/10.1186/s43045-020-00078-1

Kielhofner, G., Dobria, L., Forsyth, K., & Kramer, J. (2010). The occupational self assessment: Stability and the ability to detect change over time. *OTJR: Occupation, Participation and Health*, 30(1), 11–19. https://doi.org/10.3928/15394492-20091214-03

Kimball, J. G. (2023). Sensory modulation challenges: One missing piece in the diagnosis and treatment of veterans with PTSD. *Occupational Therapy in Mental Health*, 39(3), 314–331. https://doi.org/10.1080/0164212X.2022.2131695

Kimball, J. G., Cao, L., & Draleau, K. S. (2018). Efficacy of the Wilbarger Therapressure Program™ to modulate arousal in women with post-traumatic stress disorder: A pilot study using salivary cortisol and behavioral measures. *Occupational Therapy in Mental Health*, 34(1), 86–101. https://doi.org/10.1080/0164212X.2017.1376243

King, L. J. (1974). A sensory-integrative approach to schizophrenia. *American Journal of Occupational Therapy*, 28(9), 529–536.

Kinnealey, M., & Fuiek, M. (1999). The relationship between sensory defensiveness, anxiety, depression and perception of pain in adults. *Occupational Therapy International*, 6(3), 195–206. https://doi.org/10.1002/oti.97

Kiresuk, T. J., & Sherman, R. E. (1968). Goal attainment scaling: A general method for evaluating comprehensive community mental health programs. *Community Mental Health Journal*, 4, 443–453. https://doi.org/10.1007/BF01530764

Kiresuk, T. J., Smith, A., & Cardillo, J. E. (1994). *Goal Attainment Scaling: Applications, Theory and Measurement*. Erlbaum.

Kirsh, B., Martin, L., Hultqvist, J., & Ecklund, M. (2019). Occupational therapy interventions in mental health: A literature review in search of evidence. *Occupational Therapy in Mental Health*, 35(2), 109–156. https://doi.org/10.1080/0164212X.2019.1588832

Kontaris, I., East, B. S., & Wilson, D. A. (2020). Behavioral and neurobiological convergence of odor, mood and emotion: A review. *Frontiers in Behavioral Neuroscience*, 14, article 35. https://doi.org/10.3389/fnbeh.2020.00035

Koomar, J. (2009). Trauma and attachment-informed sensory integration assessment and intervention. *Sensory Integration Special Interest Section Quarterly*, 32(4), 1–4.

Kramer, J., Kielhofner, G., Lee, S. W., Ashpole, E., & Castle, L. (2009). Utility of the Model of Human Occupation Screening Tool for detecting client change. *Occupational Therapy in Mental Health*, 25(2), 181–191. https://doi.org/10.1080/01642120902859261

Krause-Utz, A., Frost, R., Chatzaki, E., Winter, D., Schmahl, C., & Elzinga, B. M. (2021). Dissociation in borderline personality disorder: Recent experimental, neurobiological studies, and implications for future research and treatment. *Current Psychiatry Reports*, 23(37). https://doi.org/10.1007/s11920-021-01246-8

Lad, M., Sedley, W., & Griffiths, T. D. (2022). Sensory loss and risk of dementia. *Neuroscientist*, 30(2). https://doi.org/10.1177/10738584221126090

Lane, S. J. (2020a). Structure and Function of the Sensory Systems. In A. C. Bundy & S. J. Lane (eds), *Sensory Integration: Theory and Practice* (3rd ed.) (pp. 58–114). F. A. Davis.

Lane, S. J. (2020b). Sensory Modulation Functions and Disorders. In A. C. Bundy & S. J. Lane (eds), *Sensory Integration: Theory and Practice* (3rd ed.) (pp. 151–180). F. A. Davis.

Lane, S. J., Mailloux, Z., Schoen, S., Bundy, A., et al. (2019). Neural foundations of Ayres Sensory Integration®. *Brain Sciences*, 9(7), 153. https://doi.org/10.3390/brainsci9070153

Law, M. Baptiste, S., Carswell, A., McColl, M. A., Polatajko, H., & Pollock, N. (1998). *Canadian Occupational Performance Measure* (3rd ed.). CAOT Publications ACE.

Law, M., Baptiste, S., Carswell, A., McColl, M. A., Polatajko, H., & Pollock, N. (1994a). *The Canadian Occupational Performance Measure* (2nd ed.). CAOT Publications.

Law, M., Polatajko, H., Pollock, N., McColl, M. A., Carswell, A., & Baptiste, S. (1994b). Pilot testing of the Canadian Occupational Performance Measure: Clinical and Measurement Issues. *Canadian Journal of Occupational Therapy*, 61, 191–197. https://doi.org/10.1177/000841749406100403

Lawrence, C., & Mcauley, S. (2023). Eating Disorders. In W. Bryant, J. Creek & N. Pastow (eds), *Occupational Therapy and Mental Health* (6th ed.) (pp. 511–531). Elsevier.

Lee, S., & Harris, M. (2010). The development of an effective occupational therapy assessment and treatment pathway for women with a diagnosis of borderline personality disorder on an inpatient setting. *British Journal of Occupational Therapy*, 73(11), 559–563. https://doi.org/10.4276/030802210X12892992239396

Lehrner, A., Daskalakis, N., & Yehuda, R. (2016). Cortisol and the Hypothalamic–Pituitary–Adrenal axis in PTSD. In J. D. Bremner (ed.), *Posttraumatic Stress Disorder: From Neurobiology to Treatment* (pp. 265-290). Wiley-Blackwell.

Lei, Y., & Wang, J. (2017). The effect of proprioceptive acuity variability on motor adaptation in older adults. *Experimental Brain Research*, 236, 599–608. https://doi.org/10.1007/s00221-017-5150-x

Lindberg, M. H., Samuelsson, M., Perseius, K. I., & Björkdahl, A. (2019). The experiences of patients in using sensory rooms in psychiatric inpatient care. *International Journal of Mental Health Nursing*, 28(4), 930–939. https://doi.org/10.1111/inm.12593

Linehan, M. M. (1993). *Skills Training Manual for Treating Borderline Personality Disorder*. Guilford Press.

Lins, L., & Carvalho, F. M. (2016). SF-36 total score as a single measure of health-related quality of life: Scoping review. *SAGE Open Med*, 4:2050312116671725. https://doi.org/10.1177/2050312116671725

Lipskaya-Velikovsky, L., Bar-Shalita, T., & Bart, O. (2015). Sensory modulation and daily-life participation in people with schizophrenia. *Comprehensive Psychiatry*, 58, 130–137. https://doi.org/10.1016/j.comppsych.2014.12.009

Livingston, G., Huntley, J., Sommerlad, A., Ames, D., et al. (2020). Dementia prevention, intervention, and care: 2020 report of the Lancet Commission. *The Lancet*, 396 (10248), 413–446. https://doi.org/10.1016/S0140-6736(20)30367-6

Löffler, A., Foell, J., & Bekrater-Bodmann, R. (2018). Interoception and its interaction with self, other, and emotion processing: Implications for the understanding of psychosocial deficits in borderline personality disorder. *Current Psychiatry Reports, 20*(28). https://doi.org/10.1007/s11920-018-0890-2

Löffler, A., Kleindienst, N., Neukel, C., Bekrater-Bodmann, R., & Flor, H. (2022). Pleasant touch perception in borderline personality disorder and its relationship with disturbed body representation. *Borderline Personality Disorder and Emotion Dysregulation, 9*(1), 1–16. https://doi.org/10.1186/s40479-021-00176-4

Logan, B., Jegatheesan, D., Viecelli, A., Pascoe, E., & Hubbard, R. (2022). Goal attainment scaling as an outcome measure for randomised controlled trials: A scoping review. *BMJ Open, 12*(7), e063061. https://doi.org/10.1136/bmjopen-2022-063061

Lorusso, L. N., & Bosch, S. J. (2018). Impact of multisensory environments on behavior for people with dementia: A systematic literature review. *The Gerontologist, 58*(3), e168–e179. https://doi.org/10.1093/geront/gnw168

Lowey, R. L., Corey, S., Amirfathi, F., Dabit, S., et al. (2019). Childhood trauma and clinical high risk for psychosis. *Schizophrenia Research, 205*, 10–14. https://doi.org/10.1016/j.schres.2018.05.003

Lundy-Eckman, L. (2013). *Neuroscience: Fundamentals for Rehabilitation* (4th ed.). Elsevier.

Lynch, H., & Moore, A. (2016). Play as an occupation in occupational therapy. *British Journal of Occupational Therapy, 79*(9), 519–520. https://doi.org/10.1177/0308022616664540

Ma, W. Y., Tian, M. J., Yao, Q., Li, Q., et al. (2022). Neuroimaging alterations in dementia with Lewy bodies and neuroimaging differences between dementia with Lewy bodies and Alzheimer's disease: An activation likelihood estimation meta-analysis. *CNS Neuroscience and Therapeutics, 28*(2), 183–205. https://doi.org/10.1111/cns.13775

Mahler, K. (2019). *The Interoception Curriculum: A Step-By-Step Framework for Developing Mindful Self-Regulation*. Mahler Autism Services.

Mahler, K. (2017). *Interoception: The Eighth Sensory System*. AAPC Publishing.

Mailloux, Z., Parham, D., Smith-Roley, S., Ruzzano, L., & Schaaf, R. C. (2018). Introduction to the Evaluation in Ayres Sensory Integration® (EASI). *American Journal of Occupational Therapy, 72*(1). https://doi.org/10.5014/ajot.2018.028241

Malejko, K., Huss, A., Schönfeldt-Lecuona, C., Braun, M., & Graf, H. (2020). Emotional components of pain perception in borderline personality disorder and major depression – a repetitive peripheral magnetic stimulation (rPMS) study. *Brain Sciences, 10*(12), 905. https://doi.org/10.3390/brainsci10120905

Malejko, K., Neff, D., Brown, R. C., Plener, P. L., et al. (2018). Somatosensory stimulus intensity encoding in borderline personality disorder. *Frontiers in Psychology, 9*. https://doi.org/10.3389/fpsyg.2018.01853

Matson, R., Barnes-Brown, V., & Stonall, R. (2024). The impact of childhood trauma on sensory processing and connected motor planning and skills: A scoping review. *Journal of Child and Adolescent Trauma, 17*, 447–456. https://doi.org/10.1007/s40653-023-00598-y

Matson, R., Kriakous, S., & Stinson, M. (2021). The experiences of women with a diagnosis of borderline personality disorder (BPD) using sensory modulation approaches in an inpatient mental health rehabilitation setting. *Occupational Therapy in Mental Health, 37*(4), 311–331. https://doi.org/10.1080/0164212X.2021.1933674

May-Benson, T. (2017). *Influence of Complex Trauma and Attachment on Praxis and Play Concerns in Children*. https://thespiralfoundation.org/product/influence-of-complex-trauma-and-attachment-on-praxis-and-play-concerns-in-children

May-Benson, T. (2015). *Adolescent/Adult Sensory History*. Spiral Foundation.

May-Benson, T., & Easterbrooks-Dick, O. (2016). *Adult/Adolescent Sensory History: Short Report*. Spiral Foundation. https://thespiralfoundation.org/adult-adolescent-sensory-history-2

McGreevy, S., & Boland, P. (2022). Touch: An integrative review of a somatosensory approach to the treatment of adults with symptoms of post-traumatic stress disorder. *European Journal of Integrative Medicine, 54*. https://doi.org/10.1016/j.eujim.2022.102168

McGreevy, S., & Bolland, P. (2020). Sensory-based interventions with adult and adolescent trauma survivors: An integrative review of the occupational therapy literature. *Irish Journal of Occupational Therapy, 48*(1), 31–54. https://doi.org/10.1108/IJOT-10-2019-0014

McIntosh, D. N., Miller, L. J., & Shyu, V. (1999). Development and Validation of the Short Sensory Profile. In W. Dunn (ed.), *Sensory Profile: User's Manual* (pp. 59–73). Psychological Corporation.

Mehling, W. E., Price, C., Daubenmier, J. J., Acree, M., Bartmess, E., & Stewart, A. (2018). *Multidimensional Assessment of Interoceptive Awareness*. https://osher.ucsf.edu/research/maia

Migeot, J. A., Duran-Aniotz, C. A., Signorelli, C. M., Piguet, O., & Ibanez, A. (2022). A predictive coding framework of allostatic-interoceptive overload in frontotemporal dementia. *Trends in Neurosciences, 45*(11), 838–853. https://doi.org/10.1016/j.tins.2022.08.005

Mikulska, J., Juszczyk, G., Gawrońska-Grzywacz, M., & Herbet, M. (2021). HPA axis in the pathomechanism of depression and schizophrenia: New therapeutic strategies based on its participation. *Brain Sciences*, 11(10). https://doi.org/10.3390/brainsci11101298

Miller, L. J., & Parham, L. D. (2020). Distilling Sensory Integration Theory for Use: Making Sense of the Complexity. In A. C. Bundy & S. J. Lane (eds), *Sensory Integration Theory and Practice* (3rd ed.) (pp. 338-349). F. A. Davis.

Miller, L. J., Reisman, J. E., Mcintosh, D. N., & Simon, J. (2001). An Ecological Model of Sensory Modulation: Performance of Children with Fragile X Syndrome, Autistic Disorder, Attention-Deficit/Hyperactivity Disorder, and Sensory Modulation Dysfunction. In S. Smith Roley, E. I. Blanche & R. Schaaf (eds), *Sensory Integration with Diverse Populations* (pp. 57-88). Pro-ed.

Miller, L. J., Schoen, S. A., Mulligan, S., & Sullivan, J. (2017). Identification of sensory processing and integration symptom clusters: A preliminary study. *Occupational Therapy International*. https://doi.org/10.1155/2017/2876080

Mulligan, S., Schoen, S., Miller, L., Valdez, A., Wiggins, A., Hartford, B., & Rixon, A. (date of publication pending). Initial Studies of Validity of the Sensory Processing 3-Dimensions Scale. *Physical & Occupational Therapy In Pediatrics*, 39(1), 94-106. https://doi.org/10.1080/01942638.2018.1434717

Moore, K. M., & Henry, A. D. (2002). Treatment of adult psychiatric patients using the Wilbarger protocol. *Occupational Therapy in Mental Health*, 18(1), 43-63. https://doi.org/10.1300/J004v18n01_03

Moore, K. M., & McCraith, D. (1998). *Sensory-Based Treatment: The Missing Piece in DBT* [Paper presentation]. The Massachusetts Association for Occupational Therapy (MAOT) conference, Boston, MA.

Mukherjee, A., Biswas, A., Roy, A., Biswas, S., et al. (2017). Behavioural and psychological symptoms of dementia: Correlates and impact on caregiver distress. *Dementia and Geriatric Cognitive Disorders*, 7, 354-365. https://doi.org/10.1159/000481568

Munro, C., Randell, L., & Lawrie, S. M. (2016). An integrative bio-psycho-social theory of anorexia nervosa. *Clinical Psychology & Psychotherapy*, 24(1), 1-21. https://doi.org/10.1002/cpp.2047

Murphy, F., Nasa, A., Cullinane, D., Gazzaz, A., et al. (2022). Childhood trauma, the HPA axis and psychiatric illnesses: A targeted literature synthesis. *Frontiers in Psychiatry*, 13. https://doi.org/10.3389/fpsyt.2022.748372

National Disability Authority (2015). Universal Design Guidelines: Dementia Friendly Dwellings. https://universaldesign.ie/built-environment/housing/dementia-friendly-dwellings

National Institute for Health and Care Excellence (NICE) (2022). *Depression in Adults: Treatment and Management* [NG222]. www.nice.org.uk/guidance/ng222

National Institute for Health and Care Excellence (NICE) (2018). *Dementia: Assessment, Management and Support for People Living With Dementia and Their Carers* [NG97]. www.nice.org.uk/guidance/ng97/resources/dementia-assessment-management-and-support-for-people-living-with-dementia-and-their-carers-pdf-1837760199109

National Institute for Health and Care Excellence (NICE) (2014). *Bipolar Disorder: Assessment and Management* [CG185]. www.nice.org.uk/guidance/cg185

National Institute on Ageing (2023). How the Aging Brain Affects Thinking. www.nia.nih.gov/health/brain-health/how-aging-brain-affects-thinking

NHS (2023). Symptoms - Schizophrenia. www.nhs.uk/mental-health/conditions/schizophrenia/symptoms

Ogden, P. (2021). The different impact of trauma and relational stress on physiology, posture, and movement: Implications for treatment. *European Journal of Trauma and Dissociation*, 5(4). https://doi.org/10.1016/j.ejtd.2020.100172

Ogden, P., & Fischer, J. (2015). *Sensorimotor Psychotherapy: Interventions for Trauma and Attachment*. W. W. Norton & Company.

Ogden, P., Minton, K., & Pain, C. (2006). *Trauma and the Body*. W. W. Norton & Company.

Ohno, K., Tomori, K., Sawada, T., Seike, Y., Yaguchi, A., & Kobayashi, R. (2021). Measurement properties of the Canadian Occupational Performance Measure: A systematic review. *American Journal of Occupational Therapy*, 75(6). https://doi.org/10.5014/ajot.2021.041699

O'Neill, A., D'Souza, A., Samson, A. C., Carballedo, A., Kerskens, C., & Frodl, T. (2015). Dysregulation between emotion and theory of mind networks in borderline personality disorder. *Psychiatry Research: Neuroimaging*, 231(1), 25-32. https://doi.org/10.1016/j.pscychresns.2014.11.002

Osborne, K. J., Kraus, B., Curran, T., Earls, H., & Mittal, V. A. (2022). An event-related potential investigation of early visual processing deficits during face perception in youth at clinical high risk for psychosis. *Schizophrenia Bulletin*, 48(1), 90-99. https://doi.org/10.1093/schbul/sbab068

O'Sullivan, J., & Fitzgibbon, C. (2018). *Sensory Modulation Resource Manual*. Sensory Modulation Brisbane.

Özata Değerli, M. N., & Altuntaş, O. (2023). Are behavioral and psychological symptoms of dementia related to sensory processing? *Applied Neuropsychology: Adult*, 1–7. https://doi.org/10.1080/23279095.2023.2232067

Palmquist, E., Larsson, M., Olofsson, J. K., Seubert, J., Bäckman, L., & Laukka, E. J. (2020). A prospective study on risk factors for olfactory dysfunction in aging. *Journals of Gerontology: Series A*, 75(3), 603–610. https://doi.org/10.1093/gerona/glz265

Paquet, A., Calvet, B., Lacroix, A., & Girard, M. (2022). Sensory processing in depression: Assessment and intervention perspective. *Clinical Psychology and Psychotherapy*, 29(5), 1567–1579. https://doi.org/10.1002/cpp.2785

Parham, L. D., & Ecker, C. L. (2007). *Sensory Processing Measure (SPM)*. Pearson.

Parham, L. D., Ecker, C. L., Kuhaneck, H., Henry, D. A., & Glennon, T. J. (2021). *Sensory Processing Measure, Second Edition (SPM-2)*. Western Psychological Services.

Parham, L. D., Roush, S., Downing, D. T., Michael, P. G., & McFarlane, W. R. (2019). Sensory characteristics of youth at clinical high risk for psychosis. *Early Intervention in Psychiatry*, 13(2), 264–271. https://doi.org/10.1111/eip.12475

Parham, L. D., Smith-Roley, S., May-Benson, T. A., Koomar, J., et al. (2011). Development of a fidelity measure for research on the effectiveness of the Ayres Sensory Integration® intervention. *American Journal of Occupational Therapy*, 65, 133–142. https://doi.org/10.5014/ajot.2011.000745

Parker, G., Paterson, A., Romano, M., & Graham, R. (2017). Altered sensory phenomena experienced in bipolar disorder. *American Journal of Psychiatry*, 174(12), 1146–1150. https://doi.org/10.1176/appi.ajp.2017.16121379

Parkinson, S., Cooper, J., de las Heras de Pablom, C. G., & Forsyth, K. (2014). Measuring the effectiveness of interventions when occupational performance is severely impaired. *British Journal of Occupational Therapy*, 77(2), 78–81. https://doi.org/10.4276/030802214X13916969447155

Parkinson, S., Forsyth, K., & Kielhofner, G. (2006). *The Model of Human Occupation Screening Tool (Version 2.0)*. Model of Human Occupation Clearinghouse.

Pearson Education (2019). *Adolescent/Adult Sensory Profile: Technical Report*. www.pearsonassessments.com/content/dam/school/global/clinical/us/assets/sensory-profile/aasp-technical-report.pdf

Peng, W., Jia, Z., Huang, X., Lui, S., Kuang, W., et al. (2019). Brain structural abnormalities in emotional regulation and sensory processing regions associated with anxious depression. *Progress in Neuro-Psychopharmacology and Biological Psychiatry*, 94. https://doi.org/10.1016/j.pnpbp.2019.109676

Perry, B. D. (2009). Examining childhood maltreatment through a neurodevelopmental lens: Clinical applications of the neurosequential model of therapeutics. *Journal of Loss and Trauma*, 14, 240–255. https://doi.org/10.1080/15325020903004350

Perry, B. D. (2006). The Neurosequential Model of Therapeutics: Applying Principles of Neuroscience to Clinical Work with Traumatized and Maltreated Children. In N. Boyd Webb (ed.), *Working With Traumatized Youth in Child Welfare* (pp. 27–52). New York.

Perry, B. D., & Szalavitz, M. (2017). *The Boy Who Was Raised as a Dog* (3rd ed.). Basic Books.

Pezzoli, S., & Venneri, A. (2021). Neuroimaging Findings in Patients with Hallucinations: Evidence from Neurodegenerative and Psychiatric Conditions. In R. A. Dierckx, A. Otte, E. F. J. de Vries, A. van Waarde and I. E. Sommer (eds), *PET and SPECT in Psychiatry* (pp. 555–587).

Pfeiffer, B., Brusilovskiy, E., Bauer, J., & Salzer, M. S. (2014). Sensory processing, participation, and recovery in adults with serious mental illnesses. *Psychiatric Rehabilitation Journal*, 37(4), 289–296. https://doi.org/10.1037/prj0000099

Pfeiffer, B., & Kinnealey, M. (2003). Treatment of sensory defensiveness in adults. *Occupational Therapy International*, 10(3), 175–184. https://doi.org/10.1002/oti.184

Pohl, P. S., Dunn, W., & Brown, C. (2003). The role of sensory processing in the everyday lives of older adults. *OTJR: Occupation, Participation and Health*, 23(3), 99–106. https://doi.org/10.1177/153944920302300303

Porges, S. (2015). Making the world safe for our children: Down-regulating defence and up-regulating social engagement to 'optimise' the human experience. *Children Australia*, 40(2), 114–123. https://doi.org/10.1017/cha.2015.12

Porges, S. (2009). Examining child maltreatment through a neurodevelopmental lens: Clinical applications of the neurosequential model of therapeutics. *Journal of Loss and Trauma*, 14, 240–255. https://doi.org/10.1080/15325020903004350

Porter, C., Palmier-Claus, J., Branitsky, A., Mansell, W., Warwick, H., & Varese, F. (2020). Childhood adversity and borderline personality disorder: A meta-analysis. *Acta Psychiatrica Scandinavica*, 141(1), 6–20. https://doi.org/10.1111/acps.13118

Potkins, D., Myint, P., Bannister, C., Tadros, G., et al. (2003). Language impairment in dementia: Impact on symptoms and care needs in residential homes. *International Journal of Geriatric Psychiatry*, 18(11), 1002–1006. https://doi.org/10.1002/gps.1002

Puckett, L., Grayeb, D., Khatri, V., Cass, K., & Mehler, P. (2021). A comprehensive review of complications and new findings associated with anorexia nervosa. *Journal of Clinical Medicine*, 10(12). https://doi.org/10.3390/jcm10122555

Punski-Hoogervorst, J. L., Avital, A., & Engel-Yeger, B. (2023). Challenges in basic and instrumental activities of daily living among adults with posttraumatic stress disorder: A scoping review. *Occupational Therapy in Mental Health*, 39(2), 184–210. https://doi.org/10.1080/0164212X.2022.2094523

Puppala, G. K., Gorthi, S. P., Chandran, V., & Gundabolu, G. (2021). Frontotemporal dementia – current concepts. *Neurology India*, 69(5), 1144–1152. https://doi.org/10.4103/0028-3886.329593

Quesnel, D. A., Cooper, M., Fernandez-del-Valle, M., Reilly, A., & Calogero, R. M. (2023). Medical and physiological complications of exercise for individuals with an eating disorder: A narrative review. *Journal of Eating Disorders*, 11, 3. https://doi.org/10.1186/s40337-022-00685-9

Raihani, N. J., & Bell, V. (2019). An evolutionary perspective on paranoia. *Nature Human Behaviour*, 3(2), 114–121. https://doi.org/10.1038/s41562-018-0495-0

Ramsay, I. S., Schallmo, M. P., Biagianti, B., Fisher, M., Vinogradov, S., & Sponheim, S. R. (2020). Deficits in auditory and visual sensory discrimination reflect a genetic liability for psychosis and predict disruptions in global cognitive functioning. *Frontiers in Psychiatry*, 11. https://doi.org/10.3389/fpsyt.2020.00638

Rhodus, E. K., Hunter, E. G., Rowles, G. D., Bardach, S. H., et al. (2022). Sensory processing abnormalities in community-dwelling older adults with cognitive impairment: A mixed methods study. *Gerontology and Geriatric Medicine*, 8, 1–11. https://doi.org/10.1177/23337214211068290

Richard, L. F., & Knis-Matthews, L. (2010). Are we really client-centered? Using the Canadian Occupational Performance Measure to see how the client's goals connect with the goals of the occupational therapist. *Occupational Therapy in Mental Health*, 26(1), 51–66. https://doi.org/10.1080/01642120903515292

Richter, E., & Oetter, P. (1990). Environmental Matrices for Sensory Integrative Treatment. In S. Murrill (ed.), *Environment: Implications for Occupational Therapy Practice. A Sensory Integrative Perspective.* AOTA.

Rieke, E. F., & Anderson, D. (2009). Adolescent/Adult Sensory Profile and obsessive–compulsive disorder. *American Journal of Occupational Therapy*, 63(2), 138–145. https://doi.org/10.5014/ajot.63.2.138

Rinne-Albers, M. A., Nienke Pannekoek, J., Van Hoof, M., Van Lang, N. D., et al. (2017). Anterior cingulate cortex grey matter volume abnormalities in adolescents with PTSD after childhood sexual abuse. *European Neuropsychopharmacology*, 27(11), 1163–1171. https://doi.org/10.1016/j.euroneuro.2017.08.432

Riva, G., & Dakanalis, A. (2018). Altered processing and integration of multisensory bodily representations and signals in eating disorders: A possible path toward the understanding of their underlying causes. *Frontiers in Human Neuroscience*, 12(49). https://doi.org/10.3389/fnhum.2018.00049

Rosenthal, M. Z., Ahn, R., & Geiger, P. J. (2011). Reactivity to sensations in borderline personality disorder: A preliminary study. *Journal of Personality Disorders*, 25(5), 715. https://doi.org/10.1521/pedi.2011.25.5.715

Royal College of Occupational Therapists (2023). *Weighted Blankets for Children and Adults: A Guide for Occupational Therapists.* https://www.rcot.co.uk/latest-news/rcot-weighted-blankets-guide-occupational-therapists

Royal College of Occupational Therapists (2021). *Professional Standards for Occupational Therapy Practice, Conduct and Ethics.* Royal College of Occupational Therapists.

Royal College of Occupational Therapists (2018). *Embracing Risk; Enabling Choice: Guidance for Occupational Therapists* (3rd ed.). Royal College of Occupational Therapists. www.rcot.co.uk/practice-resources/rcot-publications/downloads/embracing-risk

Royal College of Speech and Language Therapists (2019). *Key Questions to Ask When Selecting Outcome Measures: A Checklist for Allied Health Professionals.* www.rcslt.org/wp-content/uploads/media/docs/selecting-outcome-measures.pdf

Safe Wards (2023). Calm Down Methods. www.safewards.net/interventions/calm-down-methods

Sakaki, M., Murayama, K., Izuma, K., Aoki, R., et al. (2024). Motivated with joy or anxiety: Does approach-avoidance goal framing elicit differential reward-network activation in the brain? *Cognitive, Affective, and Behavioural Neuroscience*, 24, 469–490. https://doi.org/10.3758/s13415-024-01154-3

Salamone, P. C., Legaz, A., Sedeño, L., Moguilner, S., et al. (2021). Interoception primes emotional processing: Multimodal evidence from neurodegeneration. *Journal of Neuroscience*, 41(19), 4276–4292. https://doi.org/10.1523/JNEUROSCI.2578-20.2021

Sanchis-Asensi, A., Triviño-Juárez, J. M., Sanchis-Almiñana, H., and Romero-Ayuso, D. (2022). Relationship between sensory profile and self-perceived quality of life in people with schizophrenia: An exploratory study. *Occupational Therapy in Mental Health*, 1–19. https://doi.org/10.1080/0164212X.2022.2125925

Sanford, J., Law, M., Swanson, L., & Guyatt, G. (1994). Assessing clinically important change as an outcome of rehabilitation in older adults. *Proceedings of the American Society of Aging*. San Francisco, CA.

Saure, E., Lepistö-Paisley, T., Raevuori, A., & Laasonen, M. (2022). Atypical sensory processing is associated with lower body mass index and increased eating disturbance in individuals with anorexia nervosa. *Frontiers in Psychiatry, 13*. https://doi.org/10.3389/fpsyt.2022.850594

Scanlan, J. N., & Novak, T. (2015). Sensory approaches in mental health: A scoping review. *Australian Occupational Therapy Journal, 62*, 277–285. https://doi.org/10.1111/1440-1630.12224

Schaaf, R. C., Benevides, T., Mailloux, Z., Faller, P., et al. (2014). An intervention for sensory difficulties in children with autism: A randomized trial. *Journal of Autism and Developmental Disorders, 44*, 1493–1506. https://doi.org/10.1007/s10803-013-1983-8

Schaaf, R. C., & Mailloux, Z. (2015). *Clinician's Guide for Implementing Ayres Sensory Integration®: Promoting Participation for Children With Autism*. AOTA.

Schmitz, M., Bertsch, K., Löffler, A., Steinmann, S., Herpetz, S. C., & Bekrater-Bodmann, R. (2021). Body connection mediates the relationship between traumatic childhood experiences and impaired emotion regulation in borderline personality disorder. *Borderline Personality Disorder and Emotion Regulation, 8*(17). https://doi.org/10.1186/s40479-021-00157-7

Schoen, S. A., Lane, S. J., Mailloux, Z., May-Benson, T., et al. (2019). A systematic review of Ayres Sensory Integration intervention for children with autism. *Autism Research, 12*(1), 6–19. https://doi.org/10.1002/aur.2046

Schoen, S. A., Miller, L. J., & Sullivan, J. C. (2014). Measurement in sensory modulation: The Sensory Processing Scale Assessment. *American Journal of Occupational Therapy, 68*(5), 522–530. https://doi.org/10.5014/ajot.2014.012377

Selby, E. A., Harnedy, L. E., Hiner, M., & Kim, J. (2022). Developmental and momentary dynamics in the onset and maintenance of nonsuicidal self-injurious behavior and borderline personality disorder. *Current Psychiatry Reports, 24*, 897–909. https://doi.org/10.1007/s11920-022-01396-3

Sensory Attachment Intervention (no date). What Is SAI? www.sensoryattachmentintervention.com

Serafini, G., Gonda, X., Canepa, G., Pompili, M., et al. (2017). Extreme sensory processing patterns show a complex association with depression, and impulsivity, alexithymia, and hopelessness. *Journal of Affective Disorders, 210*, 249–257. https://doi.org/10.1016/j.jad.2016.12.019

Serafini, G., Gonda, X., Pompili, M., Rihmer, Z., Amore, M., & Engel-Yeger, B. (2016). The relationship between sensory processing patterns, alexithymia, traumatic childhood experiences, and quality of life among patients with unipolar and bipolar disorders. *Child Abuse and Neglect, 62*, 39–50. https://doi.org/10.1016/j.chiabu.2016.09.013

Shaffer Jr, J. J., Johnson, C. P., Fiedorowicz, J. G., Christensen, G. E., Wemmie, J. A., & Magnotta, V. A. (2018). Impaired sensory processing measured by functional MRI in bipolar disorder manic and depressed mood states. *Brain Imaging and Behavior, 12*(3), 837–847. https://doi.org/10.1007/s11682-017-9741-8

Siegel, D. (1999). *The Developing Mind*. Guilford Publications.

Sim, L., & Peterson, C. B. (2021). The peril and promise of sensitivity in eating disorders. *International Journal of Eating Disorders, 54*(11), 2046–2056. https://doi.org/10.1002/eat.23606

Singh, K. (2016). Nutrient and stress management. *Journal of Nutrition and Food Sciences, 6*(4), 528. http://dx.doi.org/10.4172/2155-9600.1000528

Sleep Foundation (2023). Sleep Diary. www.sleepfoundation.org/sleep-diary

Smith, T. O., Lockey, D., Johnson, H., Rice, L., Heard, J., & Irving, L. (2023). Pain management for people with dementia: A cross-setting systematic review and meta-ethnography. *British Journal of Pain, 17*(1), 6–22. https://doi.org/10.1177/20494637221119588

Sørlie, C., Cowan, M., Chacksfield, J., Vaughan, E., & Atler, K. E. (2020). Occupation-focused assessment in eating disorders: Preliminary utility. *Occupational Therapy in Mental Health, 36*(2), 145–161. https://doi.org/10.1080/0164212X.2020.1719271

Spangler, N. W. (2011). Mood Disorders. In C. Brown & V. C. Stoffel (eds), *Occupational Therapy in Mental Health: A Vision for Participation* (pp. 182–196). F. A. Davis.

Spitzer, R. L., Kroenke, K., Williams, J. B., & Löwe, B. (2006). A brief measure for assessing generalized anxiety disorder: The GAD-7. *Archives of Internal Medicine, 166*(10), 1092–1097. https://doi.org/10.1001/archinte.166.10.1092

Spooner, R. K., Taylor, B. K., L'Heureux, E., Schantell, M., et al. (2021). Stress-induced aberrations in sensory processing predict worse cognitive outcomes in healthy aging adults. *Aging, 18*, 13–16. https://doi.org/10.18632%2Faging.203433

Stackhouse, T. M., Burke, H. K., Hacker, C. G., Burke, L. M., et al. (2023). Integrated occupational therapy camp for children with regulation/sensory processing differences: Preliminary evaluation. *Canadian Journal of Occupational Therapy, 90*(1), 25–33. https://doi.org/10.1177/00084174221129941

Strøm, B. S., Ytrehus, S., & Grov, E. K. (2016). Sensory stimulation for persons with dementia: A review of the literature. *Journal of Clinical Nursing, 25*(13–14), 1805–1834. https://doi.org/10.1111/jocn.13169

Su, C.-T., Ng, H.-S., Yang, A.-L., & Lin, C.-Y. (2014). Psychometric evaluation of the Short Form 36 Health Survey (SF-36) and the World Health Organization Quality of Life Scale Brief Version (WHO-QOL-BREF) for patients with schizophrenia. *Psychological Assessment, 26*(3), 980–989. https://psycnet.apa.org/doi/10.1037/a0036764

Sutton, D., Wilson, M., Van Kessel, K., & Vanderpyl, J. (2013). Optimizing arousal to manage aggression: A pilot study of sensory modulation. *International Journal of Mental Health Nursing, 22*(6), 500–511. https://doi.org/10.1111/inm.12010

Swenor, B. K., Wang, J., Varadaraj, V., Rosano, C., et al. (2019). Vision impairment and cognitive outcomes in older adults: The Health ABC Study. *Journals of Gerontology: Series A Biological Sciences and Medical Sciences, 74*, 1454–1460. https://doi.org/10.1093/gerona/gly244

Tahami Monfared, A. A., Byrnes, M. J., White, L. A., & Zhang, Q. (2022). Alzheimer's disease: Epidemiology and clinical progression. *Neurology and Therapy, 11*(2), 553–569.

Teicher, M. H., & Samson, J. A. (2016). Annual research review: Enduring neurobiological effects of childhood abuse and neglect. *Journal of Child Psychology and Psychiatry, 57*(3), 241–266. https://doi.org/10.1111/jcpp.12507

Tennant, R., Hiller, L., Fishwick, R., Platt, S., et al. (2007). The Warwick-Edinburgh Mental Well-Being Scale (WEMWBS): Development and UK validation. *Health and Quality of Life Outcomes, 5*, Article 63. https://doi.org/10.1186/1477-7525-5-63

Thomas, E. C., Read, H., Neumann, N., Zagorac, S., et al. (2022). Implementation of occupational therapy within early intervention in psychosis services: Results from a national survey. *Early Intervention in Psychiatry, 17*(7), 652–661. https://doi.org/10.1111/eip.13359

Thomas, J. J., Lawson, E. A., Micali, N., Misra, M., Deckersbach, T., & Eddy, K. T. (2017). Avoidant/restrictive food intake disorder: A three-dimensional model of neurobiology with implications for etiology and treatment. *Current Psychiatry Reports, 19*, 1–9. https://doi.org/10.1007/s11920-017-0795-5

Toussaint, A., Hüsing, P., Gumz, A., Wingenfeld, K., et al. (2020). Sensitivity to change and minimal clinically important difference of the 7-item Generalized Anxiety Disorder Questionnaire (GAD-7). *Journal of Affective Disorders, 265*, 395–401. https://doi.org/10.1016/j.jad.2020.01.032

Turner-Stokes, L. (2009). *Goal Attainment Scaling in Rehabilitation: A Practical Guide*. www.kcl.ac.uk/nmpc/assets/rehab/gas-goal-attainment-scaling-in-rehabilitation-a-practical-guide.pdf

Utley, E., Pettit, K., & Robertson, D. (1983). Southern California Postrotary Nystagmus Test: Adult normative data. *Occupational Therapy in Mental Health, 3*(4), 29–33. https://doi.org/10.1300/J004v03n04_03

Van der Kolk, B. (2015). *The Body Keeps the Score: Brain, Mind and Body in the Healing of Trauma*. Penguin.

Van der Kolk, B. (2005). Developmental trauma disorder: Toward a rational diagnosis for children with complex trauma histories. *Psychiatric Annals, 35*(5), 401–408. https://doi.org/10.3928/00485713-20050501-06

Varese, F., Smeets, F., Drukker, M., Lieverse, R., et al. (2012). Childhood adversities increase the risk of psychosis: A meta-analysis of patient-control, prospective- and cross-sectional cohort studies. *Schizophrenia Bulletin, 38*(4), 661–671. https://doi.org/10.1093/schbul/sbs050

Vaughan, S., Failla, M. D., Poole, H. M., Forshaw, M. J., et al. (2019). Pain processing in psychiatric conditions: A systematic review. *Review of General Psychology, 23*(3), 336–358. https://doi.org/10.1177/1089268019842771

Wallis, K., Sutton, D., & Bassett, S. (2018). Sensory modulation for people with anxiety in a community mental health setting. *Occupational Therapy in Mental Health, 34*(2), 122–137. https://doi.org/10.1080/0164212X.2017.1363681

Ware, J. E., & Sherbourne, C. D. (1992). The MOS 36-Item Short-Form Health Survey (SF-36): 1. Conceptual framework and item selection. *Medical Care, 30*(6), 473–483.

Warner, E., Koomar, J., Lary, B., & Cook, A. (2013). Can the body change the score? Application of sensory modulation principles in the treatment of traumatized adolescents in residential settings. *Journal of Family Violence, 28*(7), 729–738. https://doi.org/10.1007/s10896-013-9535-8

Watling, R., & Hauer, S. (2015). Effectiveness of Ayres Sensory Integration® and sensory-based interventions for people with autism spectrum disorder: A systematic review. *American Journal of Occupational Therapy*, 69(5), 1–12. https://doi.org/10.5014/ajot.2015.018051

Wiglesworth, S., & Farnworth, L. (2016). An exploration of the use of a sensory room in a forensic mental health setting: Staff and patient perspectives. *Occupational Therapy International*, 23(3), 255–264. https://doi.org/10.1002/oti.1428

Wei, Y., & Van Someren, E. (2020). Interoception relates to sleep and sleep disorders. *Current Opinion in Behavioral Sciences*, 33, 1–7. https://doi.org/10.1016/j.cobeha.2019.11.008

Wilbarger, J. L., & Wilbarger, P. L. (2020). Wilbarger Approach to Treating Sensory Defensiveness. In A. C. Bundy & S. J. Lane (eds), *Sensory Integration Theory and Practice* (3rd ed.) (pp. 426–431). F. A. Davis.

Wilbarger, P., & Wilbarger, J. L. (1991). *Sensory Defensiveness in Children Aged 2–12: An Intervention Guide for Parents and Other Caretakers*. Therapro.

Williamson, P., & Ennals, P. (2020). Making sense of it together: Youth & families co-create sensory modulation assessment and intervention in community mental health settings to optimise daily life. *Australian Occupational Therapy Journal*, 67(5), 458–469. https://doi.org/10.1111/1440-1630.12681

Windsor, M., Smith Roley, S., & Szklut, S. (2001). Assessment of Sensory Integration and Praxis. In S. Smith-Roley, E. I. Blanche & R. C. Schaaf (eds), *Understanding the Nature of Sensory Integration With Diverse Populations* (pp. 215–246). Pro-ed.

World Health Organization (WHO) (2021). Dementia. www.who.int/news-room/facts-in-pictures/detail/dementia

World Health Organization (WHO) (2012). *The World Health Organization Quality of Life (WHOQOL)*. www.who.int/publications/i/item/WHO-HIS-HSI-Rev.2012.03

Wright, L., Meredith, P., & Bennett, S. (2022). Sensory approaches in psychiatric units: Patterns and influences of use in one Australian health region. *Australian Occupational Therapy Journal*, 69(5), 559–573. https://doi.org/10.1111/1440-1630.12813

Wright, S. (2020). The Clinical Relevance of Sensory Processing Sensitivity: Observing Correlations with Depression and Anxiety [Unpublished doctoral thesis]. Chicago School of Professional Psychology.

Yamamotova, A., Bulant, J., Bocek, V., & Papezova, H. (2017). Dissatisfaction with own body makes patients with eating disorders more sensitive to pain. *Journal of Pain Research*, 10, 1667–1675. http://dx.doi.org/10.2147/JPR.S133425

Yochman, A., & Pat-Horenczyk, R. (2020). Sensory modulation in children exposed to continuous traumatic stress. *Journal of Child and Adolescent Trauma*, 13, 93–102. https://doi.org/10.1007/s40653-019-00254-4

Zaree, M., Hassani Mehraban, A., Lajevardi, L., Saneii, S., Pashazadeh Azari, Z., & Mohammadian Rasnani, F. (2023). Translation, reliability and validity of Persian version of Adolescent/Adult Sensory Profile in dementia. *Applied Neuropsychology: Adult*, 30(1), 1–7. https://doi.org/10.1080/23279095.2021.1904927

Zhang, W., Low, L. F., Schwenk, M., Mills, N., Gwynn, J. D., & Clemson, L. (2019). Review of gait, cognition, and fall risks with implications for fall prevention in older adults with dementia. *Dementia and Geriatric Cognitive Disorders*, 48(1–2), 17–29. https://doi.org/10.1159/000504340

Zhou, H. Y., Yang, H. X., Cui, X. L., Shi, L. J., et al. (2020). Self-reported sensory responsiveness patterns in typically-developing and early-onset schizophrenia adolescents: Its relationship with schizotypal and autistic traits. *Journal of Psychiatric Research*, 131, 255–262. https://doi.org/10.1016/j.jpsychires.2020.10.002

Zhou, S., Su, S., Hong, A., Yang, C., et al. (2022). Abnormal functional connectivity of brain regions associated with fear network model in panic disorder. *World Journal of Biological Psychiatry*, 23(10), 764–772. https://doi.org/10.1080/15622975.2022.2038389

Zigmund, A. S., & Snaith, R. P. (1983). The Hospital Anxiety and Depression Scale. *Acta Psychiatrics Scandinavica*, 67(6), 361–370. https://doi.org/10.1111/j.1600-0447.1983.tb09716.x

Zilbershlag, Y., Ravitz-Ron, K., & Engel-Yeger, B. (2023). The role of altered sensory processing and its association with participation in daily activities and quality of life among older adults in the community. *Occupational Therapy in Healthcare*, 37(2), 230–247. https://doi.org/10.1080/07380577.2022.2025552

Subject Index

Adolescent/Adult Sensory Profile (AASP) 115–7, 120–1, 135
Adult/Adolescent Sensory History (ASH) 117–9, 135, 185–6
affective and anxiety disorders
  alterations in sensory processing 73–6
  amygdala and 82–3, 83f
  arousal increasing strategies 87–9
  arousal reduction strategies 85–7
  assessment approaches 83–4, 193–4
  auditory input differences 76
  auditory strategies 87, 88–9
  bipolar disorder 73
  case study (Remi) 89–90
  depression 73, 74, 75
  impact on access to regulation 74–5, 74f
  impact of sensory processing on functioning 78–80
  medication 80
  neurological threshold 73–5
  panic attacks 82
  proprioceptive strategies 86, 88
  sensory lens on anxiety 81–3, 83f
  sensory support plans 84–5
  sleep issues 80–1
  strategies/approaches 84–9
  tactile input differences 75
  tactile strategies 86–7, 88
  taste and olfactory strategies 86, 88
  vestibular strategies 86, 88
  visual processing differences 76
  visual strategies 87, 88
ageing, and sensory loss 128
agoraphobia 79
Alzheimer's disease 91, 94, 95t, 97, 98
amygdala
  and affective and anxiety disorders 82–3, 83f
  and psychotic disorders 19–20, 20f

anorexia nervosa 45, 46–8, 47, 48, 49, 49–50
anxiety *see* affective and anxiety disorders
aromatherapy oils 28, 40, 54, 69, 104, 152, 158
assessment approaches
  affective and anxiety disorders 83–4
  borderline personality disorder (BPD) 37–9
  dementia 101–2
  eating disorders 51–3
  psychotic disorders 24–5
  PTSD/trauma 65–7
Assessment of Motor and Process Skills (AMPS) 124–5
assessment/assessment tools
  36-Item Short Form Survey Instrument (SF-36) 193
  Adolescent/Adult Sensory Profile (AASP) 115–7, 120–1, 135
  Adult/Adolescent Sensory History (ASH) 117–9, 135, 185–6
  and ageing/sensory loss 128
  Assessment of Motor and Process Skills (AMPS) 124–5
  auditory discrimination 131
  auditory modulation 132
  Canadian Occupational Performance Measure (COPM) 191–2
  capturing occupational changes 187–9
  capturing sensory changes 185
  clinical observations 102, 123, 125–6, 129–32, 136, 187
  cognitive ability changes and 128–9
  Evaluation in Ayres Sensory Integration (EASI) 122, 136, 187
  Generalized Anxiety Disorder Questionnaire (GAD-7) 194
  getting supporting information from others 129

SUBJECT INDEX

goal attainment scaling (GAS) 188-9
Hospital Anxiety and Depression
  Scale (HADS) 194
identifying appropriate 114-5
interoceptive discrimination 131
Model of Human Occupation
  Exploratory Level Outcome
  Ratings (MOHO-ExpLOR) 191
Model of Human Occupation
  Screening Tool (MOHOST) 190
Multidimensional Assessment
  of Interoceptive Awareness,
  Version 2 (MAIA-2) 120
non-standardized 121
Occupational Self-Assessment
  (OSA) 190-1
overview 184-5
performance-based assessments 121-2
proprioceptive discrimination 130
reflective tools 195
self-report and carer report
  assessments 115-20
Sensory Integration and Praxis
  Test (SIPT) 122-3, 187
Sensory Processing 3-Dimensions
  Scale (SP3D) 114, 124
Sensory Processing Measure, Second
  Edition (SPM-2) 119-20, 135, 186
sensory-informed functional assessments
  and observations 129-32
sleep scales 194
specific mental health conditions 127
Structured Observations of
  Sensory Integration - Motor
  (SOSI-M) 123, 136
tactile discrimination 130-1
tactile modulation 132
vestibular discrimination 130
vestibular modulation 132
visual discrimination 131
visual modulation 132
Warwick-Edinburgh Mental Wellbeing
  Scale (WEMWBS) 193
WHOQOL-100 and WHOQOL-
  BREF 192-3
auditory processing differences
  affective and anxiety disorders 76
  borderline personality disorder (BPD)
  34
  signs of 131, 132
auditory strategies
  affective and anxiety disorders 87, 88-9

dementia 106, 107
  in group programme 208-10
  overview 154-5
avoidant/restrictive food intake
  disorder (ARFID) 46
Ayres Clinical Observations 125
Ayres Sensory Integration (ASI) therapy
  background 168-9
  client-led activities 176-7
  equipment 170-4, 181-2
  mentoring 178-9
  overview 143-4, 145t
  playfulness in 175-6
  process elements 174-7
  safe space 174
  structural elements 170-4
  suitable spaces for 177-8, 180-2
  swings 170-1, 181
Ayres Sensory Integration Fidelity Measure
  (ASIFM) 144, 168, 169, 170, 174

binge eating disorder 45-6
bipolar disorder 73
body awareness strategies
  borderline personality
    disorder (BPD) 41-2
  eating disorders 55-6
  psychotic disorders 27
borderline personality disorder (BPD)
  alterations in sensory processing 32-5
  altered pain thresholds 36-7
  assessment approaches 37-9
  auditory processing differences 34
  body awareness strategies 41-2
  case study (Aoife) 42-4
  childhood trauma and 32
  hypothalamic-pituitary-adrenal
    (HPA) axis dysregulation 33
  impact of sensory processing
    on functioning 35-6
  interoceptive processing differences 34
  intervention approaches 39
  neurological threshold 32-4, 33f
  overview 31
  praxis and motor planning 35
  proactive strategies 40-1
  proprioceptive input differences 34
  reactive strategies 40
  safety plans 39-40
  self-harm 36-7, 39
  strategies/approaches 39-42
  structures of the brain affected 33f

binge eating disorder *cont.*
   tactile input differences 34
   thalamus role 32
bulimia nervosa 45, 47

'calm down methods' 148
Canadian Occupational Performance
   Measure (COPM) 191–2
client-led approach 11, 13, 176–7
clinical observations 102, 123,
   125–6, 129–32, 136, 187
cognitive functioning
   changes in ability 128–9
   psychotic disorders and 23

deep pressure touch 54–5, 66, 68, 153
dementia
   aberrant motor behaviour 92
   alterations in sensory processing 92–8
   Alzheimer's disease 91, 94, 95t, 97, 98
   arousal increasing strategies 106–7
   arousal reduction strategies 104–6
   assessment approaches 101–2
   auditory strategies 106, 107
   behavioural and psychological
      symptoms of 92
   brain areas impacted 95–6, 95t
   carer/family involvement 101–2
   case study (Dana) 111–2
   communication strategies 108–9
   design principles (dementia-
      friendly) 99–100
   frontotemporal dementia 91, 95t, 97
   impact of sensory processing
      on functioning 98–100
   interoceptive processing 97
   intervention approaches 102–3
   Lewy body dementia 91, 95t, 98
   memory and reminiscence therapy 100
   motor planning 98
   multi-sensory environments (MSEs) 108
   neurological threshold 93–6
   olfactory processing 96–7
   overview 91–2
   personal care strategies 109–10
   proprioceptive strategies 104, 106
   risk factors 96
   sensory support plans 103
   tactile input differences 97
   tactile strategies 105–6, 107
   taste and olfactory strategies 104, 107
   vascular dementia 91
   vestibular strategies 104, 106
   visual strategies 106, 107
   vs healthy ageing process 93
depression 73, 74, 75
dialectical behavioural therapy 38
dissociation 69–70
distraction strategies 28

eating disorders
   anorexia nervosa 45, 46–8,
      47, 48, 49, 49–50
   assessment approaches 51–3
   binge eating disorder 45–6
   body awareness strategies 55–6
   bulimia nervosa 45, 47
   case study (Joanne) 57–8
   exercise and movement 51
   hypothalamic–pituitary–adrenal (HPA)
      axis dysregulation 47–8, 48f
   impact of sensory processing
      on functioning 50
   interoceptive difficulties 47, 56
   interoceptive processing 49
   intervention approaches 51–3
   neurological threshold 46–8, 48f
   overview 45–6
   regulation support 54–5
   sensory systems differences 48–50
   strategies/approaches 53–6
   tactile input differences 49
   visual input differences 49–50
environmental adaptations 141–2, 142t, 166
Evaluation in Ayres Sensory Integration
   (EASI) 122, 136, 187
expert (client as own) 11, 176–7

fidget items 27, 28, 41, 109, 158, 210
first episode psychosis 16
flashbacks 64–5
frontotemporal dementia 91, 95t, 97
functioning (impact of sensory
   processing on)
   affective and anxiety disorders 78–80
   borderline personality disorder (BPD) 35–6
   dementia 98–100
   eating disorders 50
   psychotic disorders 22–3
PTSD/trauma 64

Generalized Anxiety Disorder
   Questionnaire (GAD-7) 194

goal attainment scaling (GAS) 188–9
goal setting 133–4, 184–5, 188–9
grounding strategies (psychotic disorders) 26–7
group programme 201–17
gym ball 40, 69, 126, 150, 158, 171, 172

hallucinations 23–4
hippocampus (and psychotic disorders) 19–20, 20f
Hospital Anxiety and Depression Scale (HADS) 194
hyper-vigilance 64–5, 69
hypothalamic–pituitary–adrenal (HPA) axis dysregulation
    affective and anxiety disorders 76–8, 77f
    borderline personality disorder (BPD) 33
    eating disorders 47–8, 48f
    psychotic disorders 18
    PTSD/trauma 62

Interoception Curriculum 165
interoception strategies in group programme 214–5
interoceptive processing differences
    assessing 120
    borderline personality disorder (BPD) 34
    dementia 97
    eating disorders 49, 56
    Sensory Profile Interoception (SPI) scale 52
    signs of 131–2
intervention approaches
    borderline personality disorder (BPD) 39
    dementia 102–3
    eating disorders 51–3
    psychotic disorders 25–6
    PTSD/trauma 65–7

levels of intervention
    overview 138
    sensory strategies 139–41
    summary of 144, 145t
Lewy body dementia 91, 95t, 98
linear vestibular input 150

medication
    affective and anxiety disorders 80
    side effects 127
mentoring 178–9
Model of Human Occupation Exploratory Level Outcome Ratings (MOHO-ExpLOR) 191
Model of Human Occupation Screening Tool (MOHOST) 190
motor planning
    borderline personality disorder (BPD) 35
    dementia 98
    psychotic disorders 21–2
    PTSD/trauma 63
movement strategies in group programme 212–4
multi-sensory environments (MSEs) 108, 145t
Multidimensional Assessment of Interoceptive Awareness, Version 2 (MAIA-2) 120
music as a strategy 155

neurological thresholds
    affective and anxiety disorders 73–5
    borderline personality disorder (BPD) 32–4, 33f
    dementia 93–6
    psychotic disorders 17–8, 18–20f
    PTSD/trauma 60–2, 61f

Observations Based on Sensory Integration Theory 102, 136
observations (clinical) 102, 123, 125–6, 129–32, 136, 187
Occupational Self-Assessment (OSA) 190–1
olfactory strategies
    affective and anxiety disorders 86, 88
    borderline personality disorder 40
    dementia 96–7, 104, 107
    eating disorders 54
    overview 151–2
    psychotic disorders 26
    PTSD/trauma 69

pain thresholds (altered) 36–7
panic attacks 82
peripheral nervous system (PNS) changes 128
person-centred focus 11, 13, 176–7
playfulness 175–6
praxis
    borderline personality disorder (BPD) 35
    PTSD/trauma 63
    Sensory Integration and Praxis Test (SIPT) 122–3, 187

proactive strategies (for borderline
personality disorder) 40–1
proprioceptive input differences
borderline personality disorder (BPD) 34
signs of 130
proprioceptive strategies
affective and anxiety disorders 86, 88
ASI therapy 171–3
dementia 104, 106
overview 151
psychotic disorders
alterations in sensory processing 17–22
amygdala and 19–20, 20f
arousal/concentration strategies 27
assessment approaches 24–5
auditory processing 20–1
body awareness strategies 27
case study (Jaxon) 28–9
categories of 16
differences in specific sensory
systems 20–1
distraction strategies 28
grounding strategies 26–7
hallucinations 23–4
hippocampus and 19–20, 20f
hypothalamic-pituitary-adrenal
(HPA) axis dysregulation 18
impact of sensory processing
on functioning 22–3
intervention approaches 25–6
medication 127
motor planning 21–2
neurological thresholds 17–8
phases of 16
positive and negative symptoms 15
prefrontal cortex and 19–20, 20f
schizoaffective disorder 16
strategies/approaches 26–8
thalamus disconnectivity 18–20, 20f
underlying neuroscience
considerations 18–20, 20f
visual processing 20–1
see also schizophrenia
PTSD/trauma
alterations in sensory processing 60–3
assessment/intervention
considerations 65–7
bottom-up approach 65
and BPD 32
brain areas impacted by 61–2, 61f
case study (Sofia) 70–1
deep pressure touch strategies 68

dissociation (strategies for) 69–70
flashbacks 64–5
fluctuating pattern in 60, 65
hyper-vigilance 64–5, 69
hypothalamic–pituitary–adrenal
(HPA) axis dysregulation 62
impact of sensory processing
on functioning 64
nature of (and sensory impact) 63
neurological threshold 60–2, 61f
overview 59–60
praxis and motor planning 63
and prefrontal cortex 61
proprioceptive strategies 67–8
and schizophrenia 18
strategies/approaches 67–70
tactile input differences 62
vestibular strategies 69
vestibular system differences 62

quality of life measures 192–3

reactive strategies (for borderline
personality disorder) 40
reflective tools 195
regulation
access to 74–5, 74f
support (eating disorders) 54–5
reminiscence therapy 100
risk assessment 156–8
rotational vestibular input 150

Safe Exercise at Every Stage
(SEES) guidance 53
safety
sense of 66, 67–8
supporting feelings of 67–8
safety plans (borderline personality
disorder) 39–40
schizophrenia
brain areas impacted 20f
and childhood trauma 18
identifying 16
motor planning 21–2
neurological thresholds 17
thalamus role 19
self-harm 36–7, 39
sensory assessment report template 196–8
sensory attachment intervention
(SAI) 165–6
sensory diets 149

sensory dissonance 141
sensory group programme 201–17
Sensory Integration and Praxis
    Test (SIPT) 122–3, 187
sensory kits 155–7
Sensory Patterns Questionnaire 140
sensory plans 84–5, 103, 149, 156–7
Sensory Processing 3-Dimensions
    Scale (SP3D) 114, 124
sensory processing
    bidirectional relationship in
        12, 139–40, 139f
    foundational to everything 10
    implications for occupational needs 12–4
Sensory Processing Measure Second
    Edition (SPM-2) 119–20, 135, 186
sensory rooms 143, 163–5
sensory strategies
    as 'calm down methods' 148
    developing a sensory kit 155–7
    evidence for using 148
    harmful strategies 147
    overview 139–41, 147–8
sensory support plan template 199–200
sleep issues 80–1
sleep scales 194
SMART goals 133
Snoezelen rooms 163–5
SNS response 77–8
social functioning (psychotic
    disorders and) 22
social isolation (affective and
    anxiety disorders and) 79
spaces (for ASI sessions) 177–8
Structured Observations of Sensory
    Integration – Motor (SOSI-M) 123, 136

tactile input differences
    affective and anxiety disorders 75
    borderline personality disorder (BPD) 34
    dementia 97
    eating disorders 49
    PTSD/trauma 62
    signs of 130, 130–1, 132
tactile strategies
    affective and anxiety disorders 86–7, 88
    ASI therapy 173–4
    deep pressure touch 54–5, 66, 68, 153
    dementia 105–6, 107
    in group programme 210–2
    light touch 153–4
    overview 152–3
taste and olfactory strategies
    affective and anxiety disorders 86, 88
    dementia 104, 107
    overview 151–2
thalamus role
    borderline personality disorder 32
    psychotic disorders 18–20, 20f
    schizophrenia 19
Therapeutic Listening programme
    142, 145t, 162–3
Theraputty 151, 156, 158
36-Item Short Form Survey
    Instrument (SF-36) 193
training session 218–31
trauma see PTSD/trauma

vascular dementia 91
vestibular strategies
    affective and anxiety disorders 86, 88
    dementia 104, 106
    overview 150
    PTSD/trauma 69
    swings 170–3, 181
vestibular system differences
    (PTSD/trauma) 62
visual processing differences
    affective and anxiety disorders 76
    eating disorders 49–50
    signs of 131, 132
visual strategies
    affective and anxiety disorders 87, 88
    dementia 106, 107
    in group programme 206–8
    overview 154

Warwick-Edinburgh Mental Wellbeing
    Scale (WEMWBS) 193
weighted blanket/shawl 42, 54, 68, 153, 157
weights 27, 42, 86, 151, 212, 213
WHOQOL-100 and WHOQOL-BREF 192–3
Wilbarger approach 142, 145t, 160–2

window of tolerance 76–8, 77f, 202–4

Author Index

Abi-Dargham, A. 21, 23
Acevedo, B. P. 48
Alhaj, H. A. 148
Ali, T. 127
Allee-Herndon, K. A. 175
Altuntaş, O. 92, 93, 94
Alves, J. 95, 96, 97, 99
American Psychiatric
 Association 15, 16,
 31, 36, 45, 46, 59
Anderson, D. 115
Anticevic, A. 19, 20, 23
Asher, A. V. 122, 125
Australian Health Ministers'
 Advisory Council 148
Ayres, A. J. 10, 35, 114, 122,
 123, 152, 162, 187
Azuela, G. 148

Back, S. N. 34
Bailliard, A. 13, 22,
 99, 141, 166
Balaji, G. K. 162
Barel, E. 77
Barker, M. S. 118
Baron, K. 111, 190
Bear, M. 18, 19, 32, 33, 77, 82
Behrman, S. 91
Bell, K. 46, 48, 49
Bell, V. 127
Bertsch, K. 34
Bhreathnach, E. 165, 166
Bilek, E. 32
Birba, A. 97, 120
Bitran, S. 74
Blanche, E. I. 51, 102,
 114, 117, 123, 125,
 136, 151, 187
Bolland, P. 59, 62, 64, 65

Borghammer, P. 95
Bosch, J. 192
Bosch, S. J. 99
Brand-Gothelf, A.
 46, 47, 48, 49
Breckenridge, J. 184
Brockmeyer, T. 46
Brooks, R. 190, 191
Brown, A. 138
Brown, C. 17, 19, 24, 32, 37,
 47, 52, 57, 60, 66, 70,
 75, 83, 94, 102, 111, 114,
 115, 116, 135, 143, 185
Brown, J. 16
Brown, S. 34, 38
Brown, T. 49, 186
Bugajska, K. 190, 191
Bundy, A. C. 10, 33,
 35, 38, 41, 49, 53,
 66, 93, 174, 175
Buysse, D. J. 194

Carter, O. 21
Carter, S. 51
Carvalho, F. M. 193
Cerejeira, J. 92
Cermak, S. 35, 38, 41, 67, 123
Chalmers, A. 163, 164
Champagne, T. 23, 59, 64,
 92, 109, 111, 113, 121, 149
Cheng, C. H. 76
Cheong, L. S. 73, 74, 79
Cherian, K. 18
Chung, J. C. C. 93, 94, 108
Clifford, C. 175
Cobbaert, L. 47, 49, 50, 56
Colle, L. 34, 36
Collier, L. 96, 98, 99,
 102, 108, 143, 163

Cooper, J. 191
Correia, C. 93, 128
Costantini, M. 20
Cox, A. 63
Cozolino, L. 61, 77, 169
Crail-Melendez, D.
 18, 19, 20, 23
Craswell, G. 148, 164
Crittenden, P. 165
Cromwell, R. L. 19
Crowe, J. 96
Cusic, E. 96, 98

Dakanalis, A. 50
Dark, E. 51
de Beurs, E. 193
De Lecea, L. 81
Dean, E. E. 73
Dementia UK 91
Dempsey, A. 11
Dimitriou, T. 92, 103
Dintica, C. S. 96
Dobinson, A. 53
Dorn, E. 163
Doroud, N. 143
Drews, E. 33
Duhn, L. 152
Duncan, E. A. 184
Dunn, W. 10, 17, 24, 32,
 37, 47, 52, 57, 60, 66,
 70, 73, 75, 79, 83, 93,
 94, 102, 111, 114, 115,
 116, 120, 140, 143,
 147, 185, 228, 231

Easterbrooks-Dick,
 O. 118, 185
Ecker, C. L. 119

Elias, G. J. 82
Engel-Yeger, B. 60, 61, 62, 66, 73, 79, 80, 81, 93, 116
Ennals, P. 11
Eshkevari, E. 49, 50

Falk-Kessler, J. 17, 18, 21, 115
Farnworth, L. 163
Feinstein, J. S. 82
Feldman, R. 22
Fisher, A. G. 21, 35, 65, 98, 114, 124
Fitzgibbon, C. 39
Flasbeck, V. 34
Fletcher, P. D. 95, 96, 97
Fraser, K. 65
Freedman, R. 23
French, P. 16
Frick, S. M. 142, 162
Fuiek, M. 79

Galiana-Simal, A. 46
Gaudio, S. 46, 49, 50
Gaur, N. 162
Giannopoulou, I. 18
Gibbs, G. 195
Good, K. P. 22
Guitard, P. 175
Gunnarsson, E. C. 97

Hacker, C. 142, 162
Haig, S. 148, 163
Haigh, J. 96
Hallett, N. 148, 163
Halperin, L. 17, 18, 21, 115
Harrichan, S. 59, 61, 64, 65
Harris, M. 31
Harrison, L. A. 21, 22, 49
Hart, N. 34
Hauer, S. 168, 169
Hazelton, J. L. 120
Health and Safety Executive (HSE) 15, 16
Henry, A. D. 161
Herbert, B. M. 47, 49
Hocking, C. 13
Hofmann, S. G. 74
Holland, C. M. 59, 61, 63
Holland, J. 64
Hollands, T. 66, 139

Horga, G. 20, 23
Howard, A. R. H. 62, 63
Hsu, Y. T. 123
Hughes, S. 16, 103

Jagiellowicz, J. 80
Jakob, A. 96, 98, 102, 108
Javitt, D. C. 23
Jenkinson, P. M. 47, 49
Jones, D. 184
Jonsdottir, T. 97
Joseph, R. Y. 59, 60, 61, 62, 65

Karaca Dinç, P. 59, 60
Karssemeijer, E. G. A. 103
Kearney, B. E. 60, 62
Kennedy, J. 64
Keptner, K. M. 148
Khalsa, S. S. 82, 165
Khodabakhsh, S. 73, 74, 79
Khodarahimi, S. 80
Khoweiled, A. A. 32
Kielhofner, G. 190, 191
Kimball, J. G. 149, 161, 162
King, L. J. 21, 22
Kinnealey, M. 79, 149, 161, 162
Kiresuk, T. J. 188
Kirsh, B. 190
Knis-Matthews, L. 192
Kontaris, I. 152
Koomar, J. 38, 61, 66, 68, 121, 153
Kramer, J. 190
Krause-Utz, A. 32

Lad, M. 91, 96, 97, 98
Landini, A. 165
Lane, S. J. 10, 34, 36, 49, 77, 78, 82, 93, 95, 97, 150, 162
Lanius, R. A. 60, 62
Law, M. 191, 192
Lawrence, C. 51
Lee, S. 31
Lehrner, A. 62, 65
Lei, Y. 93
Lindberg, M. H. 148, 163
Linehan, M. M. 38
Lins, L. 193

Lipskaya-Velikovsky, L. 17
Livingston, G. 96
Löffler, A. 34, 35
Logan, B. 188
Lorusso, L. N. 99
Lowey, R. L. 18
Lundy-Eckman, L. 32, 33
Lynch, H. 175

Ma, W. Y. 98
Mcauley, S. 51
McCraith, D. 38
McGreevy, S. 59, 62, 64, 65
McIntosh, D. N. 63
Mahler, K. 56, 120, 165
Mailloux, Z. 11, 122, 136, 168, 169, 170, 174, 176, 178, 184, 187, 188
Malejko, K. 32, 37
Matson, R. 39, 59, 63, 143, 148, 164
May-Benson, T. 24, 35, 38, 41, 59, 61, 63, 66, 67, 84, 102, 114, 117, 118, 127, 135, 151, 185, 197
Mehling, W. E. 84, 89, 120
Migeot, J. A. 97
Mighton, C. 96
Mikulska, J. 19, 20
Miller, L. J. 32, 93, 114, 124, 174
Moore, A. 175
Moore, K. M. 38, 161
Mukherjee, A. 92
Mulligan, S. 114, 124
Munro, C. 47
Murphy, F. 18
Murray, J. 184

National Disability Authority 99
National Institute on Ageing 128
National Institute for Health and Care Excellence (NICE) 72, 91, 100, 102
Nelson, D. L. 123
NHS 15, 16
Novak, T. 148, 164

Oetter, P. 174
Ogden, P. 60, 65, 66
Ohno, K. 192
O'Neill, A. 32
Osborne, K. J. 22
O'Sullivan, J. 39
Özata Deðerli, M. N. 92, 93, 94

Palmquist, E. 97, 99
Paquet, A. 74, 75
Parham, L. D. 17, 18, 19, 24, 67, 102, 114, 119, 122, 135, 144, 168, 169, 170, 174, 186
Parker, G. 75
Parkinson, S. 190, 191
Pat-Horenczyk, R. 62
Pearson Education 84, 102
Peng, W. 75
Perry, B. D. 35, 65, 66, 67
Peterson, C. B. 47, 48, 49
Pezzoli, S. 23
Pfeiffer, B. 17, 23, 59, 64, 149, 161, 162
Pohl, P. S. 93
Porges, S. 65, 67
Porter, C. 32
Potkins, D. 99
Puckett, L. 47
Punski-Hoogervorst, J. L. 64
Puppala, G. K. 95

Quesnel, D. A. 53

Raihani, N. J. 127
Ramsay, I. S. 20, 22
Rhodus, E. K. 94
Richard, L. F. 192
Richter, E. 174
Rieke, E. F. 115
Rinne-Albers, M. A. 61
Riva, G. 50
Rose, A. 56
Rosenthal, M. Z. 34

Royal College of Occupational Therapists 39, 54, 157, 184
Royal College of Speech and Language Therapists 188

Safe Wards 148
Sakaki, M. 134
Salamone, P. C. 120
Samson, J. A. 63
Sanchis-Asensi, A. 20, 21, 22, 24
Sanford, J. 192
Saure, E. 47, 48, 50
Scanlan, J. N. 148, 164
Schaaf, R. C. 11, 51; 125, 151, 168, 169, 170, 174, 176, 178, 184, 188
Schmitz, M. 34, 41
Schoen, S. A. 114, 124, 168
Selby, E. A. 34
Serafini, G. 60, 66, 73, 78, 115
Shaffer Jr, J. J. 76
Sherbourne, C. D. 193
Sherman, R. E. 188
Shochat, T. 81
Siegel, D. 76, 77, 202, 203, 220
Sim, L. 47, 48, 49
Sleep Foundation 194
Smith Roley, S. 122, 136
Smith, T. O. 97
Snaith, R. P. 194
Sørlie, C. 45, 51
Spangler, N. W. 74
Spitzer, R. L. 194
Spooner, R. K. 92
Stackhouse, T. M. 192
Strøm, B. S. 103
Su, C.-T. 193
Sutton, D. 163
Swenor, B. K. 99
Szalavitz, M. 66, 67
Szklut, S. 33, 35, 38, 41, 53, 66, 174, 175

Tahami Monfared, A. A. 95
Teicher, M. H. 63
Tennant, R. 193
Thomas, E. C. 23
Thomas, J. J. 46
Toussaint, A. 194
Trist, A. 148
Turner-Stokes, L. 188

Utley, E. 123

Van der Kolk, B. 59, 65, 66, 67
Van Someren, E. 97, 120
Varese, F. 18
Vaughan, S. 20
Venneri, A. 23

Wallis, K. 79, 80, 148
Wang, J. 93
Ware, J. E. 193
Warner, E. 62
Watling, R. 168, 169
Wei, Y. 97, 120
Whigham, S. C. 22
Wiglesworth, S. 163
Wilbarger, J. L. 142, 149, 160, 161
Wilbarger, P. L. 142, 149, 160, 161
Williamson, P. 11
Windsor, M. 195
World Health Organization 91, 192, 193
Wright, L. 148
Wright, S. 79

Yamamotova, A. 49, 50
Yochman, A. 62

Zaree, M. 93, 94, 95, 96
Zhang, W. 98
Zhou, H. Y. 82, 115
Zhou, S. 82
Zigmund, A. S. 194
Zilbershlag, Y. 93